A Doctor's Dictionary

Writings on Culture & Medicine

Iain Bamforth grew up in Glasgow and graduated from its medical school. He has pursued a peripatetic career as a hospital doctor, general practitioner, translator, lecturer in comparative literature, and latterly public health consultant in several developing countries, principally in Asia. His four books of poetry were joined by a fifth, *The Crossing Fee*, in 2013. His prose includes *The Body in the Library* (Verso, 2003), an account of modern medicine as told through literature; and *The Good European* (Carcanet, 2006), a collection of writings on ideas and literature in European history.

D1459004

IAIN BAMFORTH

A Doctor's Dictionary

Writings on Culture & Medicine

CARCANET

First published in Great Britain in 2015 by

Carcanet Press Limited
Alliance House
Cross Street
Manchester
M2 7AQ

www.carcanet.co.uk

We welcome your comments on our publications
Write to us at info@carcanet.co.uk

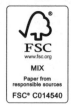

FSC
www.fsc.org
MIX
Paper from
responsible sources
FSC® C014540

A CIP catalogue record for this book is available from the British Library

ISBN 978 1 784100 56 8

The publisher acknowledges financial assistance from Arts Council England

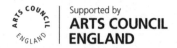

Typeset by XL Publishing Services, Exmouth
Printed and bound in England by SRP Ltd, Exeter

Hast du Verstand und ein Herz, so zeige nur eines von beiden,
Beides verdammen sie dir, zeigest du beides zugleich.

– Friedrich Hölderlin, 'Guter Rath', 1797

Contents

Preface

Anyone who decides to live on the continent (as only the British refer to it) has to expect to live part of the time in the subjunctive—the verbal mood for anything that's hypothetical or contingent. You can't hope to get by as a competent speaker of French or German (where it is called *Konjunktif*) unless you know how to enter the parallel world of things that demand someone else's participation or consent, or the special time or set of circumstances to be agreed upon before a possibility can swell into the indicative. Verbs of wishing, fearing, expressing judgement and emotion all take the subjunctive mood. The subjunctive is for people who like parentheses and extrapolations. The great Austrian novelist Robert Musil wrote an entire novel set in the subjunctive, and never emerged in the indicative to finish it.

The subjunctive exists in English too, but its presence is vestigial and barely observed. Instead we have *The Life and Opinions of Tristram Shandy, Gentleman*, Laurence Sterne's seriously funny tribute to the zigzag. His novel was once described as a congeries of 'unconnected rhapsody, rambling digression, eccentric humour, peculiar wit, petulance, pruriency and ostentation of learning'; it exhibits all those qualities, and it has also been one of the most influential European novels ever. It mocks what it loves, not least the encyclopaedic impulse; Tristram's father has a system of education 'collecting first for that purpose his own scattered thoughts, counsels, and notions, and binding them together.' This is his TRISTRA-paedia.

I took a leaf from Tristram's father's system by arranging these twenty-six essays as an abecedary of concept-terms, which is about as much order as I could give to my life. Two of these headings are not even English in origin, which is appropriate enough, and 'Posture' has a wider purchase in French, where 'être en mauvaise posture' is to be in a tricky situation. My Book of Patience includes magical and not so magical bodies, eyes and ears, nose and teeth, old-style livers and the latest pills, happiness quotients and fake doctors, Chekhov and Roget, mining towns and poison trees, Swiss sanatoria and penal colonies, and bacteria almost everywhere. Some of the concept-terms could, conceivably, have been quite different: Happiness, for instance, displaced another article on Hands, which used to be important diagnostic extensions for doctors. 'The War of Eye and Ear' was catalogued under Visions until I realised that the real concern of the essay—in spite of what Louis-Ferdinand Céline said in a 1957 interview about our species being terribly dull-witted, thick or just a drag ('extraordinaire de lourdeur')—is the increasing weightlessness of our experience, as if we were mere bundled spoors of hygiene and charisma; this made room for the Vertigo of 'Stendhal's syndrome', which could be anything from the mildest vasovagal episode to major psychotic decompensation.

My title 'A Doctor's Dictionary' is a reminder, at least to myself, that more of my professional life than I might have wanted has been spent in the precincts of weighty books, not least in France, where the unexpected difficulties of making a living as an 'omnipraticien' (general practitioner) in Strasbourg led to my becoming a scientific translator and editor. Many of these books have been dictionaries, lexicons and encyclopaedias, although with digitalisation much of their bulk and mustiness has volatilised. To be fascinated by the 'extractive industries', like the early Romantics—heightened for me by a year in a gritty but fascinating Australian mining town—is perhaps a kind of nostalgia for bodily experience, and all its effort and fatigue, now that digitisation, seemingly in league with capital, has embarked on the process of hollowing out 'all that is solid' even more drastically and purposefully than in Marx's time: there are very few jobs and professions that have not yielded to the computerisation of what they entail.

Losing touch is something that threatens us all. The implications for medicine are serious, when this ancient profession—never entirely a science and no longer quite the art it used to be, but an empirical discipline aided by, and increasingly in thrall to, technology—forgets what it owes to tact. Doctors are translators, interpreters and sign-readers, sure; but sometimes their simple presence counts for something else, as the resident asks Robert Lowell's persona in his late poem: 'We are not deep in ideas, imagination or enthusiasm—how can we help you?'

Acknowledgements

All of these pieces, with one exception, were first published in journals and periodicals, some as commissioned reviews, others as commentary pieces that I cajoled the editors into publishing. Some of them still bear the cauls of their first emergence, but generally I've attempted to coat and shoe them as literary essays, able to stand on their own while taking their place in this book's A–Z schema of things. Some first saw light as occasional pieces in the *British Journal of General Practice*, and I acknowledge a debt of gratitude to Alec Logan, its deputy editor, who for many years kept asking me to provide a feature on medicine and writing for the Christmas edition of the journal. I am also grateful to the editors of *Times Literary Supplement*, *London Review of Books*, *Medical Humanities*, *PN Review*, *Parnassus*, *Quadrant*, *The Linguist*, *Lapham's Quarterly*, *British Medical Journal*, *The Lancet* and the *Bulletin of the World Health Organization* for allowing me to develop and republish articles from their pages. 'Crise de Foie' first appeared in German translation in the weekend feuilleton of the *Süddeutsche Zeitung* thanks to the efforts of my father-in-law, Christian Schütze, who also translated it.

A number of the essays in this book constituted a good part of the manuscript *Medicine and the Imagination* submitted to the University of Glasgow in 2009 for the degree of Doctor of Letters by publication. I would like to thank Michael Schmidt and John Coyle for alerting me to the existence of a Scottish Universities by-law the terms of which were previously unknown to me, and for their encouragement, and not least that too of my external referees Kenneth Boyd and Peter Davidson, whose appraisals reassured me that I wasn't entirely on a hiding to nothing.

Thanks are also due to my helpful friend Richard Price at the British Library, and to staff at my local institute, Strasbourg's newly refurbished National and University Library (BNUS)—a magnificent Italianate edifice built in the Wilhelmine period when Strasbourg was Strassburg and second now in France in terms of its collections only to the National Library in Paris—is a precious resource for me as an expatriate writer. Further thanks are also due to colleagues and friends in medicine and the wider world, with whom I have discussed some of the issues raised in this collection at various times: Olivier Wong, Frank Slattery, Douglas Shenson, Carl Elliott, Bruce Charlton, John and Mary Gillies, Jeremy Garwood, Christopher Harvie, Christine and Richard Thayer, David Bellos, Jim Campbell, Gerald Mangan, Les Murray, Alberto Manguel, Frederic Raphael, Marjorie Farquharson, Desmond Avery, Brian Hurwitz, William Ian (Bill) Miller, Peter and Maria McCarey, as well as to my editors at Carcanet Helen Tookey and Luke Allan. I would like to thank Lewis Lapham for commissioning me to write a 'reappraisal' of *The Magic Mountain*, one of the key novels of the twentieth-century, and for Alastair Campbell and the medical ethics staff at the National University of Singapore, who allowed me to expand some of my thoughts about Hans Castorp at a meeting of their journal club. Living in Strasbourg—or 'Strasburg' as Laurence Sterne spells it in *Tristram Shandy*, where it gets a whole chapter to itself—has been to be aware of living (for twenty years now) 'far out in the centre', to purloin the title of a book by Dannie Abse: in the heart of a Europe that has no body politic. That unreality notwithstanding, my wife Cornelia was a constant presence in good and bad times, and I feel fortunate to have enjoyed the companionship of my family throughout the years covered by this book, during which my two children Felix and Claire have grown up. 'Sooner or later,' as Germain Muller, founder of the local dialect theatre *De Barabli*, noted, 'all Strasburgers end up loving Strasbourg.'

Needless to say (although it must be said), the opinions expressed in the essays engage my responsibility only.

A Doctor's Dictionary

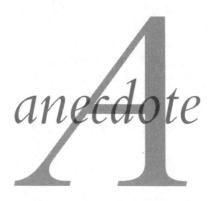

A Taste of Bitter Almonds

A STENDHAL CAPSULE

When the rotund Henri Beyle (Stendhal) dropped dead in a Paris street in 1842—'of apoplexy'—only three mourners accompanied the coffin to its resting place in the Cimetière de Montmartre: one of them was the younger writer Prosper Mérimée. Incensed by the fact that no words had been spoken at this 'pagan funeral', Mérimée wrote a short memoir of their friendship. Fact is he didn't know much about his friend other than that he had served in the Napoleonic campaigns and been a mostly indifferent diplomat in Italy, and that he was known in Paris as an occasional wit ('*homme d'esprit*') and writer with a mania for disguises; what he had read of his books didn't inspire him terribly. Perhaps because he didn't know so much about the social figure, the sketchy portrait he left, with the bare title *HB*, is a captivating one.

For a son of the post-revolutionary years like Mérimée, Beyle (born 1783) bore all the contradictory traits of a man of the previous century: 'All his life he was dominated by his imagination, and never did anything except abruptly and with enthusiasm. However, he got it into his head that he acted in conformity with reason. "One must be guided in everything by LO-GIQUE", he would say, pausing between the first syllable and the remainder of the word. But he had no patience for those whose logic differed from his own.' In fact, Stendhal was every bit a fully-fledged nineteenth-century writer of self-exploration, and he anticipated his own discovery in the twentieth (in his autobiography *La Vie de Henry Brulard* he addresses readers in 1935, not his contemporaries). Long before Flaubert and Proust, he was aware of the fitfulness and ambiguity of memory, its elusiveness when we try to snare it. Hence his famous digressive style, the comic zigzag he took from the celebrated author of *Tristram Shandy*.

Stendhal had his mnemonic devices too. As a young boy in Grenoble he had been made to take drawing lessons by his father: this got him out of the house, which he found stifling. The 175 sketches scattered throughout the text of his autobiography, showing mostly street scenes or room arrangements, reminded him of that brief moment of freedom, and served as a visual framework for his writing. Feeling that there was truth in spontaneity, he wrote quickly (his autobiography was written over four months in the winter of 1835); and although he often presents exact dates in his writings (an early talent for mathematics had allowed him at sixteen to quit the damp provincialism of Grenoble and enter the new École polytechnique in Paris), he was often slapdash in respect of actual chronology. What counted for Stendhal was the sharp, acutely characterised, discriminating account of motive or emotion. 'Love has always been for me the most important of affairs, or rather the only matter of account', he wrote, as if the ending of the sentence had only occurred to him once he had voiced the beginning. His famously mineralogical book on love talked about it in terms of a 'crystallisation'. A thinker had to be dry, clear, without illusions: a banker, he once wrote, might have the requisite character 'to make discoveries in philosophy'.

And there is his famous, light, Mozartian touch: he was as unsparing of himself as he was of others, the young provincial who hoped to cut a figure in the world and become a celebrated Don Juan even though he didn't have the physique (or, indeed, the inheritance) for it; writing his autobiography under an assumed name at fifty-three he is prepared to acknowledge that all he will be able to convey about his life of vagabondage and gallantry is the 'chasse au bonheur'—the pursuit of happiness and not the experience itself. There is no cynicism in the writing, only a serene wistfulness.

Stendhal's commitment to the brisk, discursive, associative feel of experience makes it an exhilarating experience to read his journals and travel books. Every situation in his life seems to lend itself to epigrammatic expression; and anecdotes themselves are occasions for expansive writing: in 1837–38, on leave from his consular job at Città Vecchia and visiting his own country, he dashed off a book called *Memoirs of a Tourist*. Here is a nice piece of hearsay reported in its pages which he scribbled down in Lyons, on May 19:

Three days ago Mr. Smith, an English puritan who had been living here for ten years, decided it was time to end his life. He swallowed the contents of an ounce bottle of Prussic acid. Two hours later after being very sick he was anywhere but on the point of dying, and to pass the time rolled about on the floor. His landlord, an honest cobbler, was working in his shop in the room beneath: startled by the inhabitual din and fearing that his furniture was getting a battering, he went upstairs. He knocked on the door; no reply; so he entered the room through a boarded-up door. He was aghast to see his tenant prostrate on the floor, and sent for M. Travers, well-known surgeon and friend of the sick man. The surgeon came, treated Mr. Smith, and very quickly brought him out of danger. Then he asked him: 'What the devil did you drink?'

'Some Prussic acid.'

'Impossible, six drops would have killed you in a jiffy.'

'Well, they told me it was Prussic acid.'

'Who sold it to you then?'

'The little chemist on the Quai de Saône.'

'But usually you get your prescriptions made up at Girard, your neighbour right across the street here, the best pharmacist in Lyons!'

'That's true, but the last time I bought some medicine from him, I had the impression he was overcharging me.'

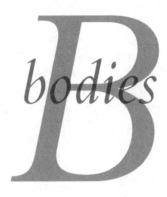

The Plastinator

ON THE ETHICS AND AESTHETICS OF A TRAVELLING
ANATOMY EXHIBITION

In 1997, in the space of four months, more than three-quarters of
a million people—the highest attendance for any post-war exhibition in Germany and more than the famous annual Dokumenta
art review in Kassel has ever attracted—queued to be admitted
to Mannheim's Regional Technical and Industrial Museum. The
exhibition attracted similar attendance figures when it moved to
Japan, reportedly receiving more than a million visitors, and to the
traditional European capitals of death, Vienna and Basel, where I
caught up with it. It is now showing in Cologne; here, too, it is
drawing in the crowds.

This is no ordinary exhibition, and not the display of fossil-
ised machine tools from Germany's long and unfinished history
of industrial achievement that might have been expected from
the museum's name. What is on show, in fact, is a collection of

about two hundred human anatomical specimens including the usual kinds of body sections, slides of diseased and healthy tissues, organs in glass cases, and so forth. These are standard objects in an exhibition of this kind. More controversial, and certainly more spectacular, are the eighteen 'plastinated' cadavers—*Ganzkörperpräparate*, or whole-body preparations.

Anatomy exhibitions have gone on the road before, though you might have to go a long way back, to the living human exhibits in the freak shows of the Victorian circus era, to find an exhibition which has aroused so much curiosity and controversy. Many of the anatomy museums in Europe's famous medical schools are either accessible to the more intrepid kind of tourist or can be consulted by appointment: I spent a long afternoon a few years ago in the mote-filled hall of the University of Montpellier's junk room, examining one of its famous series of wax impressions of syphilitic buboes and chancres from the nineteenth century. Montpellier's anatomy tradition goes back to 1315, when the body would be opened for inspection by two barbers under the instruction of a *magister* reciting the appropriate Galenic text.

It is a tradition that has been revived in several books by Frank Gonzalez-Crussi, a professor of pathology in the Children's Memorial Hospital at Northwestern University who has created a literary subgenre of his own: portrayals of the unusual and the monstrous drawn from his professional life and given a savant veneer that places them somewhere between Jorge Luis Borges and Sir Thomas Browne. In one of his essays, 'Bologna, the Learned' (in the book *Suspended Animation*, 1995) he reminds us how popular public dissections were in the fourteenth century when they were advertised by being posted in Latin, the language of the dissections, on the columns of the Archiginnasio days before the event. Public dissections became routine only at the beginning of that century. Prisoners were condemned *pro faciendo de eo notomia*—to make an anatomy of them. The cutting, rending and division of a body was a chance for the demonstrators to show the 'image of the universe' to the audience, and for learned members of the audience to engage in heated *disputatio*; it was above all an event in the social calendar. Hogarth's 'Four Stages of Cruelty' offers a very sarcastic visual commentary, in the disembowelment of poor hanged Tom Hero by a pack of doctors, on how the poor were always being held up for scrutiny by their social betters.

In those days, anatomists had to work fast to avoid the deliquescence of the body. The French surgeon Ambroise Paré (1510–90) was already recommending the use of alcohol to preserve tissues, but it was ceroplasty, or wax modelling, as developed in northern Italy—especially Florence—in the seventeenth century, that became the prized method; Gaetano Zummo's technique was brought to a fine art under the abbot Felice Fontana (1730–1805), who was able to convince artists and anatomists to work together on his waxes.

Ceroplasty was a highly skilled procedure requiring an intermixture of purified bees' wax and spermaceti, as hardener, which was then pigmented to the desired hue; special techniques such as dipping silk threads in hot wax were used to achieve the effect of fine structures—that of the lymphatic vessels or nerves for instance. Fontana's waxes were shown to great acclaim in 1780, when he was commissioned to prepare a series of obstetrical specimens for the Emperor Joseph II: these can still be seen in glass cases, as a permanent exhibit, in the palatial Josephinum in Vienna. It was hoped that they would educate Viennese doctors in the use of forceps as advocated by two pioneering Scots, Hunter and Smellie; *Tristram Shandy*, written at about the same time, descants knowingly on the optimal fulcrum placement of this new technology for use by man-midwives. Along with gross anatomy, or the study of the body as it presents itself to the naked eye, wax models were an important means of advancing the evidence of things seen when so many concepts in medicine had been hitherto deductive, reasoning from the general to the particular.

To understand the body, the body was enough—it is a very modern thought. Prior to William of Ockham, who is generally credited with giving primacy to the particular over the universal, that modern clincher 'whose body is it anyway?' would have been an inconceivable thought. Indeed, to *have* a body (a possession rather than an attribute, something like Locke's 'first property', extending its domain by assimilating what it can grasp) would have been a novel and disturbing heresy five centuries ago. Visiting Melanesia in the 1940s, the anthropologist Maurice Leenhardt was startled to be told by an elder that the Europeans had 'brought them the body'. Perhaps it was the body itself, as Durkheim suggested, that served to organise the personality. But the epis-temological strain is evident enough: after the Middle Ages, an anchorite contempt for the flesh allies itself with the Cartesian doubt that underwrites modern analytical medicine; the body loses its place in the great panpsychia of the cosmos, and the very idea of its incarnating the divine comes to seem absurdly aggrandizing. What is universal in man is now a sign.

Ceroplasty and the vascular injection of fixatives and dyes remained mainstays for teaching anatomical structure into the twentieth century. There is clearly a difference between the two methods: the first is an imitation of nature, a distancing technique, the other an attempt to preserve the corruptible body. This was not to spare the anatomist's feelings; it was to protect him from the dangers of putrefaction. The lifelikeness of prepared wax specimens can be such as to acquire a 'terrorizing' quality, as Gonzalez-Crussi puts it, although the technique met with Goethe's approval: his youthful enthusiasm for anatomy classes in Strasbourg in 1770 gave way to a suspicion that anatomists were cads of the worst kind.

On the other hand, it is probably more accurate to say that what most medical students remember of their dissection classes is not a feeling of horror at having to cut up a body but an anticli-mactic sense of how grey and shrunken the fixed cadaver is.

The illustrations from Andreas Vesalius' *De humani corporis fabrica* ranged in the museum outside the dissection room at Glasgow University were more disturbing than the cadavers inside: even when subject to terrible violence—flensed like Marsyas or hanging by a cord to keep their jaws shut—Vesalius' studies insist on comporting themselves in unmistakably lifelike ways: outrage is made complete, Baudelaire suggests in his poem 'Le Squelette Laboureur', by their being 'tricked out to look like hired hands'. Tool, image, grave: the three artifacts that take the measure of, and surpass, our ordinary human condition are assembled in the poem, yet Baudelaire's slave labourer goes on digging even after he has cut the turf for his grave, refusing to move into the immaterial. Concerning Vesalius' series, Roger Caillois remarked in his essay 'Au Cœur du Fantastique' that 'more genuine mystery crops up in such documents, in which precision is of the essence, than in the wildest inventions of Hieronymus Bosch.'

In the dissection groups of six to a table that were a feature of my days in the anatomy department of Glasgow University, imagination was stilled by the unpleasantness of the task and the pedagogic imperative: learn, learn, learn. Rote learning is drudgery: even surgeons don't need to know all the sulci, tuberosities and foramina of every bone, nor every pulley and conduit of the softer parts as detailed by Alexander Monro in his *The Anatomy of the Humane Bones* (1726). What isn't clinically important tends to be forgotten. Cynicism beckons, or you come to grief. My own enduring memory of the anatomy class is its smell, the pungent odour of formalin; it penetrated clothes and gloves, and lingered in the hair, a kind of olfactory ectoplasm from a cold place in which people no longer mattered.

Enter Professor Doktor Günther von Hagens (the 'von' is an affectation), who describes himself as 'inventor, anatomist, physician and synthetic chemist'. In the mid 1970s, at the University of Heidelberg, he developed—and patented—a new technique for preserving biological tissue called plastination. It had taken him fifteen years of experimentation with industrial solvents.

Plastination is now used by medical schools across the world for the teaching of gross anatomy. It requires tissues, or whole bodies, to be fixed in the standard way with formaldehyde or some other preservative. Specimens are then dehydrated, a process in which the fluid in the tissues is replaced with a chilled organic solvent such as acetone. The next, and central, step of the process is forced impregnation: the solvent is replaced under vacuum with a polymer, silicone or epoxy resin, producing an object which can then be manipulated in ways that were quite impossible with previous preservation techniques. The final stage involves hardening of the polymer. Tissues can be rendered pliable or hard, and with a high degree of realism. The essential organic architecture of the body is preserved, although it is now about eighty percent plastic. In all, the process takes 500–1000 working hours. It is undoubtedly an elegant technique, and produces specimens which are much more resistant to oxidation and decay than the old formalin–phenol injected bodies. Plastination can give a body 500 years of postmortem standing.

This technique, for instance, allows the skeleton to be guddled out, leaving the rest of the body, once the muscles have stiffened after absorbing the polymer, as a self-supporting 'shell'. Hagens has exploited this feature in one of his dissections on show at the Mannheim museum, where the menacing musculature of the Muscleman is displayed a step ahead of his skeleton. The skeleton has been 'shucked' of its muscles, which have been left to stand free, their bloatedness no doubt resulting from the sheer difficulty of extricating the cranium, rib cage and long bones—of outing the inner man. It is a virtuoso piece of dissection work, but the raised left arm and flailing triceps conjure up a film image: Boris Karloff as Frankenstein's monster.

Several other of the whole-body preparations in the exhibition are similarly 'exploded' to show the relationships between the internal organs, or the arterial system. Nearby, the Orthopaedic Body is decorated with twelve different prosthetic devices, and sponsored by Johnson & Johnson.

Another preparation suggests that the association between the Muscleman and Frankenstein was not fanciful: a standing figure has been defrocked of his skin which he holds in his right hand, all of a piece, with an imploring gesture. It is a direct 'quote' of the famous flayed man published by the Spanish anatomist Juan Valverde in Rome, in 1560.

Yet other dissections have 'windows' cut into the bodies at various levels indicating important internal landmarks which have to be located or avoided during surgery. One of them is a young woman with a 5-month old foetus in her uterus, the overlying rectus abdominis muscle opened in the midline to reveal the dome of the uterus pressing upwards on the intestines. Another figure, posed like a chess-player, has been pared to the ribs to show the central and peripheral nerves as they exit in pairs from the spinal column and innervate the skeletal muscles, a feat of dissection beyond the means of the traditional anatomist. The organs of a 'longitudinally expanded' preparation, which has been made to squat, shoot upwards out of the body, and are held in space by threads. 'I create space for the viewer to see the parts clearly', says Hagans, 'so that he can close the space up in his imagination.' One preparation is dissected in bands and partitions, like Dali's famous painting 'Woman with Drawers'; another is caught in the act of running, all the muscles freed from their insertions and splayed outwards. It is a dramatic portrayal of a body in motion, but it nods at the pioneering artists of the early twentieth century: the Anatomical Angel, a woman with her trapezius muscles cut and suspended like wings, in Jacques Gautier d'Agoty's atlas *Myologie complète en couleurs*, of 1746, was a fetish image for the Surrealists. Hagens' dissection is, in fact, a p(l)astiche restatement of Umberto Boccioni's visionary bronze 'Unique Forms of Continuity in Space' (1913).

Hagens is unbothered about blurring the distinction between art and dissection. He seems to thrive on it, never being seen in public himself without his Joseph Beuys fedora hat. His method of personal self-promotion stands in sharp contrast to the impersonality of his exhibits.

The Plastinator (not the *plasticator*, the epithet given to Prometheus in Ovid's *Metamorphoses*) is quick to point out that some of the best early anatomists were artists, like Leonardo da Vinci, who is thought to have dissected thirty corpses; nor is he the first anatomist to model his dissections on works of art. Honoré Fragonard's famous eighteenth century dissection of a rider on his horse, both stripped to the bone, recapitulates Dürer's 'Tod und der Reiter', and can still be seen in all its lacquered glory at the National Veterinary School at Alfort, near Paris. Frederik Ruysch (1638–1731), professor of anatomy in Amsterdam and famous for his vascular injection technique (he used a secret combination of wax, resin, talc and cinnabar which had to permeate the entire vascular system before it hardened), had five rooms in his town house at the Niewe Zijds Achterburgwal converted into a *Wunderkammer* for display of his meticulously prepared specimens and mummies. They were baroquely adorned and placed in allegorical scenes: playing a violin with a bow made of a dried artery, weeping into handkerchiefs made of mesentery or meninges, or abandoned to bewail their fate on a stage constructed out of gallstones and other body casts. Peter the Great bought the lot for the huge sum of 30,000 Dutch guilders in 1717, and had it shipped to Russia. Only half of the collection survived the journey.

Both Fragonard and Ruysch were decidedly odd characters, brooders who took their discipline to a pitch well beyond the necessary degree of scientific precision or desired illusion. In the

Mannheim exhibition catalogue, however, Hagens attempts to play down the aesthetic element, suggesting that 'the art is in the beholder's eye'.

Yet the subtitle of the exhibition itself—'die Faszination des Echten'—spells out the nature of the confusion: what status do these exhibits have? What does *real* mean here, and why should it be so fascinating? Organs and body sections aren't really that interesting unless you know what you're looking at: without the whole-body preparations, the exhibition would hardly be such a scandalous success. Heated television debates accompanied the first exhibition. Hagens was arraigned for bad taste and lack of respect for human dignity: the Mannheim theologian Johannes Reiter said, 'the person who styles human corpses as works of art no longer respects the importance of death.' Protests about its tastelessness were made by the heads of both main churches to the minister president of Baden-Württemberg, though a cool-headed sixteen-year-old pointed out in the visitors' book that the Church has a long tradition of putting its own holy mummies on display. Hagens has recruited Luther as his alias: everyone should have a chance to see the plastinated body, just as everyone should be able to read the Bible without mediation. He is 'democratizing' anatomy. 'We are not putting dead human beings on public show. The whole-body preparations on display have been anonymised and are no longer dead human beings because they are no longer the object of piety and mourning.' Article 168 of the German *Strafgesetzbuch* (on Disturbing the Peace of the Dead) has no legal force since all these former persons donated their bodies to the Institute for Plastination, thereby relinquishing their right to burial.

True enough: we don't know who these people are. We won't know their names, or the stories of their lives; even their features have been smoothed out by anatomical preparation, and the insertion of glass eyes makes them look vacuous. We may be able to guess their age, give or take a few years. Their sex is apparent. Organ deformation may give a clue as to the cause of death. That's about all that can be guessed of them in their singularity as social beings. They are empty testaments. But how can we address them except as social beings? Hagens believes that his exhibition satisfies a great longing for what he calls unadulterated originality ('unverfälschte Originalität')—a clumsy expression which might translate more simply as authenticity. What does he mean? A plastinate is not a mimetic object, like one of those glossy wax models of the seventeenth century which, by virtue of being a representation, keeps its distance. In the museum catalogue a whole-body plastinate is defined as a structural model of the cadaver (it lacks most of the water that makes up four-fifths of the human body). But an artefact can't be authentic, since an artefact is always the view of a thing, not the thing itself; nor does a cadaver have any innate structural aptitude for self-display. Hagens has to give it form by plastinating and then modelling it before hardening, a procedure ethically comparable to the partial intrusion on autonomy that occurs when a plastic surgeon reconstructs a face or body.

It is a peculiar form of playing to the gallery to insinuate, as Hagens does, that visitors to the exhibition can, in a day's viewing, locate the meaningful turnings of the very tradition which has made it possible to strip a body: a medical education is a long apprenticeship in which the discipline required to be a physician is itself re-appropriated, precept by precept. It demands participants, not onlookers.

Twenty years ago, having to dissect a body twice-weekly over nine months in the cold hall of Glasgow University's anatomy department was, as far as I was concerned, a chore; it seemed odd that a sense of medicine's embodied realism was acquired by destroying the evidence. Yet the cadaver was, in a sense, our first patient. The six of us around the table were dimly aware of the ambivalence of what we were doing: the body in front of us was no longer a human subject, but neither was it wholly in the realm of the senseless (the same cleavage attends the removal of organs from cadavers for transplantation: the sense of 'material' being cannibalised sits uncomfortably with the prospect of the 'harvested' organs sitting inside a another person). Our apprentice knowledge of anatomy had already been informed by allied disciplines, and was broadened by twice-weekly lectures on form and function delivered before we entered the cold dissection room. It was hard to appreciate then, raking someone's gizzard, that being a good doctor would entail getting beyond the old Indo-European conceptual metaphor 'knowing-is-seeing': knowing in medicine is just as much listening and touching. (Sniffing patients is not common practice these days, though diabetes can sometimes be diagnosed from a whiff of acetone in the consulting room; as for urine-tasting, it has fortunately become totally obsolete.)

But what can a 'laterally expanded' whole-body preparation convey to an observer whose only previous sense-impressions of lateral expansion have been in gore movies?

The difference between Hagens' hard plastic bodies and a simple skeleton, bereft of the conceptually rich flesh it supports, is clear enough: imagination is at work, as Hagens knows it is bound to be; which is why it is disingenuous of him to pretend that the aesthetic aspects of his preparations are only institutional and second-order, 'in the beholder's eye'.

Joseph Beuys could have told him why. Art is predicated on the exclusion of death, which obliterates the aesthetic. The only art form I can think of which meaningfully includes it—a spectator sport which culminates in an animal being put to death—is the bullfight. There the risk of failure, of being impaled on the 'bull's keen horn', is a mortal one, as noted by that restrained masochist Michel Leiris in *L'Age d'homme*; he thought it saved the torero-writer (himself) from an art of mere affectation.

The argument is one of authenticity and performance: those same strategists of liberation who had applauded the Anatomical Angel thought the process of self-discovery was a tauromachy. In fact, writing his autobiography while living his life did not elevate Leiris to the level of what Nietzsche had once called 'the dignity of a great matador'; it was to become a lifelong mortification.

The exhibition offers no new scientific discoveries: gross anatomy's heyday was long ago. The number of autopsies performed annually in hospitals has been declining for years to what pathologists regularly say are 'worryingly low levels'. Professors of anatomy these days may well be molecular biologists or biochemists, not structural anatomists.

It is ironic too that our state-of-the-art perception of the body is airier and less solid even than that of the medieval *medici*: it is a composite representation made up of vector forces, atomic energy and sound waves. The body is as permeable as it is resonant. The more we see through it, the more its substance eludes us. It is a progression that would no doubt have appealed to medieval philosophers who believed all its fleshiness was, in any case, accidental to our true essence. 'Thus we are men,' wrote Sir Thomas Browne in *Religio Medici*, 'and know not how: there is something in us that can be without us, and will be after us; though it is strange that it hath no history what it was before us, nor cannot tell how it entred in us.'

Evacuation *and* resurrection: the Greek word *exanastasis* means both—the body cannot be resurrected unless rid of its matter—or as the unshakeable Job puts it: 'And though after my skin worms destroy this body, yet in my flesh shall I see God'. Hagens' exhibition might just conceivably be a hunt for a *tertium quid*. It seems to be searching for it in the same places as the contemporary Brit Pack artists, who could well be defined as school-of-life rather than art school. It is, let it be said, a diminished life in which to go to school: reality alone counts, and reality knows nothing of representation—as if human history were an animal history.

Besides, if the body is always a symbol of society, as the anthropologist Mary Douglas insists, then society itself must be exploding at the seams. We can't expect to lay the world bare, cognitively speaking, and not feel the draught: hard knowledge after Bacon's time has meant going in fear of anatomists. Even if we were to adopt a minimal ethic with regard to the people who have donated their bodies to Hagens' institute by seeing them as in some way *performers*, the grand master of anatomical ceremony and director of the performance has an obvious responsibility not to degrade or humiliate them in their unheeding act of self-exposure.

I seem to be in a minority: most visitors to the body show actually seem to applaud the idea behind it. No objections were raised by the churches in Vienna and Basel, both of which have a long tradition of socializing their own exquisite dead. Hagens now claims to have a waiting list of a thousand 'donors', and plastination will no doubt provide an ultimate fate for some of them. Perhaps some of them are down at the gym already, shaping up for the new symbolic order.

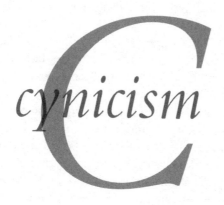

Knock! Knock!

A STUDY IN MEDICAL CYNICISM

Mundus vult decipi, ergo decipiatur
                                    – Petronius

The perfect role

In August 1923, Jules Romains (Louis Henri-Jean Farigoule), PEN
activist, friend of Stefan Zweig, and one of France's most famous
and popular writers between the wars, wrote a play in three acts
called *Knock*. It was to prove his most enduring literary creation.
In those days Romains' theatre pieces, along with those of Luigi
Pirandello and Bernard Shaw, were being staged everywhere,
which only goes to show that no literary reputation is ever entirely
vouchsafed. Indeed, the only other work for which Romains is
remembered today is his colossal 'unanimist' fiction *Les hommes
de bonne volonté*, which appeared in instalments between 1932 and
1946, when he he returned from war exile in New York and
Mexico. It runs to 8000 pages, and is published in 27 volumes. I

have yet to read it all or meet anyone who has, although Richard Cobb is right to assert, in his essay *Maigret's Paris*, that the first volume contains some finely evocative scenes of the outskirts to the French capital.

Romains first thought of asking the Comédie-Française to stage his piece. That idea came to nothing, but a copy of his play ended up in the hands of the actor Louis Jouvet who was bowled over by its 'formal perfection'. A pharmacist before he became an actor, Jouvet was for three decades one of the best-known actors of the Parisian theatre-world, a star of many classic French films including the famous *Hôtel du Nord*. With his widow's peak and suave demeanour, he looks like a svelte version of Jack Nicholson. One of his witticisms has deservedly been anthologised: 'there are performances where the public is quite without talent.'

After several rehearsals, Romains insisted that Jouvet play the character close to his own persona, without caricature—'Vous avez une occasion magnifique d'être vous-même'—but with an added touch of courtesy, sarcasm, and self-assurance. Jouvet worried that the play was going to be too 'black' to attract the public. He was wrong. On its opening night at the Comédie des Champs-Elysées on 15 December 1923, André Gide went backstage to congratulate Jouvet on his performance. From then on Jouvet *was* Knock. The play was a great success. Jouvet played the role throughout his acting life, and after the war played Knock at the Athénée no fewer than eight hundred times. Two film versions were made: one in 1933, directed by Roger Goupillières with the screenplay written by Romains himself, and a better known version, directed by Guy Lefranc, in 1951. Such was Jouvet's status that he was allowed to supervise casting. In the event, his brilliant performance proved to be the ultimate record on film of a remarkable acting career: he died on stage at the Athénée (which is now named after him) rehearsing Graham Greene's *The Power and the Glory*, just months after the film's release.

The farce and the farceur

The film opens in the early years of the twentieth century with Knock, the aspirant to a medical practice, sitting in the back of an old jalopy—the kind of automobile the French used to call a *torpédo*—with Dr Parpalaid and his wife. Knock has just purchased Dr Parpalaid's practice in the small town of Saint-Maurice, which, from the references to hilly country and the nearby presence of Lyon, would seem to indicate a sleepy hollow somewhere in the foothills of the Massif Central or the Alps. Somewhere deep in dear old France, in other words: the kind of place lost to the world that the worthy Dr Benassis decides would be suitable for his ministrations in Balzac's novel *The Country Doctor*. All the business has—unusually—been concluded in advance by letter, and Knock is exercising his right to be introduced to the clientele. Dr Parpalaid is a decent old duffer—*un homme de l'art*, as the French used to call their doctors—a man of predictable knowledge or even of 'good intent' in Romains' terms, his wife a formidable matron who seems to have far more of a head for business than her husband. Dr and Mme Parpalaid have decided, after careful consideration, to move on to better things in Lyon—she has rheumatism and her husband 'swore he would finish his career in a big city'. Urban aspirations notwithstanding, they extol the virtues of the canton to Knock: a railway far enough away for the clientele to stay put, no competitor, a chemist who doesn't try to do the doctor's job, no major overheads. Knock seems uncommonly interested in what kind of diseases his prospective clients might suffer from, and is put out to discover that the local people generally come 'only for a single consultation'. There are no regular patients: it's not like the baker or the butcher, exclaims Madame Parpalaid, who takes him for a bit wet around the ears. Knock is forty, Faust's age; though he admits to having completed his thesis only the summer before. Its title? 'On imaginary states of health', with an epigraph from Claude Bernard: *Les gens bien portants sont des malades qui s'ignorent*. Well people are sick people who don't know it yet.

This is a motto about the unwitting patient in all of us, and it turns out, ominously, to be the most telling line in the play.

There are already some subtle worrying signs about Knock. He doesn't know the church feast-days, not even Michaelmas, which is when Dr Parpalaid's patients are in the habit of paying him. (Dr Parpalaid has roguishly sold the practice just after this date, thus giving Knock grounds for accusing Parpalaid of attempting to fleece him—but when did a doctor ever buy a practice without seeing it first?) As a child he was apparently an avid and precocious reader of the information slips tucked around bottles of pills: at nine he could recite entire pharmacopoeias of side-effects. He has already been a ship's doctor, he informs Madame Parpalaid, and for the duration of the voyage had crew and passengers confined to the sick bay: only the expediency of a roster kept the ship manned and the engines running. In short, Knock has a vocation and no ordinary one at that; and he has a 'method'.

Knock arranges visits with the other members of the cabal: the teacher Mr Bernard and the pharmacist Mr Mousquet. His language is fulsome and ingratiating. He bludgeons the former with the modern horror of microbes. He describes the presentation material that will amplify the effect of his public lectures: 'All of this illustrated with superb pictures: bacilli enlarged thousands of times, typical stool patterns of typhoid patients, infected nodes, intestinal perforations, and not in black and white, but in colour: all the pinks, browns, yellows and pale greens you can imagine.' Poor Mr Bernard, who is an impressionable type, is overwhelmed, and protests that if he gets involved he won't be able to sleep himself. 'That's how it should be', retorts Knock, 'what I mean is: that's exactly the kind of fright we have to deliver. We have to shock the audience to its core [...]. Because their fatal error is to sleep the sleep of false security—then disease wakes them like a thunderclap, but it's too late, too late.'

Historically in France, pharmacists occupied the subsidiary role of *marchands-épiciers*; they were the money-hungry apothecaries and suppliers of unicorn's horn who inspired Molière to create Purgon and Fleurant. Knock flatters Mr Mousquet with talk of collegiality. A physician who can't rely on a first-class chemist is 'a general who goes into battle without artillery'. They discuss the low volume of trade generated by Dr Parpalaid, and Knock wonders 'whether he really believed in medicine'. This, for Knock, is a scandalous state of affairs when all the inhabitants of the district are potential clients.

With teacher and pharmacist now on his side, Knock engages the local odd-job man, who doubles as town-crier, to tell the country folk that consultations are to be given free of charge at the surgery on Monday mornings. When he asks the town crier what the townspeople used to call his predecessor, he discovers it was never 'Monsieur le docteur', but often a soubriquet—Ravachol. Romains is enjoying a little joke with his audience. Ravachol was a notorious anarchist in nineteenth-century France (his actual name was Kœnigstein) who ended up losing his head to the guillotine, though one of his ditties, *Le Bon Dieu dans la Merde*, was resurrected by the Situationists in the 1960s. His name marks Dr Parpalaid out as an old-fashioned believer in anarchism as against the power of capital and the State, though it has to be remembered that nineteenth-century anarchism was not irrationalist, and largely eschewed violence: it was the most serious *utopian* alternative to Marxism. It still finds some expression among French doctors who, rather than acknowledge the unwelcome fact that the medical profession needs the state to safeguard its monopoly in providing treatment, defend what they call 'liberalism' as a solid defence against the intrusions of government into private life. What had been hotly discussed issues in the 1840s were taken up again, though with a weary acerbity, after the debacle of the Great War. Romains rather vaguely defined his own philosophy of unanimism, which opposed liberalism's concept of the individual in the belief that it simply handed even more power to state bureaucracies, as 'a natural and spontaneous harmony within a group of people who share the same emotion'. His platform was a form of syndicalism. What is interesting about all this is that Kropotkin's cooperatives and Proudhon's theory of 'mutual aid'—not unlike unanimism—leaned on Darwin's law of natural selection just as much as Spencer's competitive model of evolutionary sociology and the eugenic movement that followed it, suggesting that there is no straightforward leap from scientific to political ecology. Indeed, Dr Parpalaid's anarchism—of the utopian, non-bombing, moralistic kind extolled by Tolstoy—looks mostly like a practical philosophy for smallholders.

All of this is old hat to Knock. His ideal of social organisation is a form of hygiene organised around himself as 'continual creator' and saviour. His method is finely calculated and carefully organised. He assiduously acquaints himself with the incomes of his clients. Blackboard, anatomical chart and reflecting laryngoscope are used to devastating effect in his surgery. Patients are stripped of their defences, beginning with the flimsy mantle of insouciance which has hitherto protected them from worrying about their health. 'Est-ce que ça vous chatouille, ou est-ce que ça vous gratouille', he inquires of the town crier, hilariously mangling the language, splitting hairs and echoing Hamlet all in the one phrase: 'do you have a tickling feeling, or is it more a kind of prickling?' If it's an itch the poor man thinks he has, it must be a mortal one. The Lady in Violet, a certain 'dame Pons, née demoiselle Lempoumas', gets the shock treatment: her insomnia, which Dr Parpalaid had never taken seriously—he used to tell her 'to read three pages of the civil code every evening'—may now be the result of a 'pipestem deformity' of the intracerebral circulation or perhaps even a 'sustained neuralgiform crisis of the substantia nigra'. Or perhaps, as Knock adds in an undertone, it's just a big black spider sucking on her brain.

Knock's use of 'big words' to terrorise the Lady in Violet is one of the oldest medical tricks: think of Molière's cod Latin-spouting Sganarelle in the most famous predecessor farce *le Médecin malgré lui* (1666), or the nuciform sac, a structure unknown to any anatomy textbook but wielded to good effect by the surgeon Mr Cutler Walpole in George Bernard Shaw's play *The Doctor's Dilemma* (1906). The description of Walpole in Shaw's stage-directions even resembles Jouvet's portrayal of Knock in the film: his face, according to Shaw in his stage directions, looks 'machine-made and beeswaxed; but his scrutinizing, daring eyes give it life and force. He never seems at a loss, never in doubt; one feels that if he made a mistake he would make it thoroughly and firmly...' It may be scandalous to admit it, but dissembling has long been part of medicine's therapeutic arsenal: Knock proffers big words, not for the sake of the cure but for the rather more pertinent issue of reinforcing his authority.

The nuciform sac turns up in another guise in Axel Munthe's hugely successful, if hugely self-regarding, volume of reminiscences from the same decade, *The Story of San Michele* (1929), in which he tells how, when working in a private practice, the fashionable diagnosis of colitis, invented precisely to save patients from the scalpels of surgeons like Mr Cutler Walpole, 'spread like wildfire all over Paris'. Munthe, a young Swede who qualified in Paris at the unheard-of age of twenty-two, was once called 'the most fascinating man in Europe': his persuasive bedside manner brought him a large clientele of largely wealthy patients whom he believed should be made to pay for the poorer (Knock has a system of 'means-testing' too).

Several chapters of Munthe's memoir, a best-seller in its time, are devoted to Jean-Martin Charcot, with whom he trained at the famous Paris hospital La Pitié-Salpêtrière. Patients, doctors (most notably Sigmund Freud, in 1885), and the public flocked to see the great man in action in the auditorium where his mostly but not exclusively female patients obligingly assumed, when prompted, all the dramatic postures of florid hysteria. Charcot took hypnosis seriously as a technique for healing, though the psychoanalytic movement as a whole, fearing that transference and counter-transference would contaminate the psychoanalytic method, shied away from suggestion techniques; even then, hypnosis was to stay in the bag of tricks of many psychoanalysts. Munthe's thumbnail sketch of Charcot speaks volumes for the magical function of the medicine-man in an age that proclaims itself thoroughly rational: the following passage was actually omitted from the French trans-lation of *San Michele*, presumably because its hint of diabolism failed to flatter the reputation of the Maître who had dominated French medicine for more than a generation. 'Charcot for instance was almost uncanny in the way he went straight to the root of the evil, often apparently only after a rapid glance at the patient from his cold eagle eyes.' This is a description of a magician, not a scientist.

Once Knock has made it explicit, danger is like the house dust mite: everywhere. One might call it Getting the Fear. Knock encourages the local schoolteacher, Mr Bernard, to indulge his little obsessive-compulsive tic—'Do you think, doctor... I may be a carrier of germs?' Mr Bernard's phobic reaction testifies to the power of a mystery—the invisible germ—caught in the full glare of scientific explanation. No other scientific figure stands with such emblematic clarity in republican France's sense of itself as the bacteriologist Louis Pasteur—'le bienfaiteur de l'humanité'. It was, after all, the French Revolution that gave rise to the belief that where a physician worked his cures there could be no clergy, and that illness was a matter for the common weal. The evil of profiteering doctors would disappear once equality, freedom and fraternity had borne their true fruit. Diseases would be classified; statistics collated; clinics built. Pasteur is emblematic because he embodies so well the due process of the positivist formula: theoretical research plus application of acquired knowledge makes for general well-being.

Medicine, for the nineteenth-century French, was the advance post of Progress. Such was its prestige that Zola made his novels case-histories: he anticipates one of Knock's lines in his novel *Lourdes* with the query: 'Supposing that after all there is a Power greater than that of men, higher than that of science? It is the instinctive hankering after the Lie which creates human credulity.' In Zola's literary-lab view of the world, pharmacy is on a level with semiology. While flattering Mousquet, the only chemist in town, Knock astutely promises to triple his income within a year. Besides, aren't they partners in the great fight against disease? When Mousquet points out that people have to fall ill first, Knock retorts with a policy statement: '"Fall ill"—that's an old-fashioned idea! It has been completely overhauled by modern scientific medicine. Health is a word which could just as well be struck from the dictionary. What I see are people variously affected by a various number of diseases of varying virulence. Of course, if you insist on telling them they're well, they'll be only too happy to believe you. But you're leading them on. Your only excuse can be that you already have too many patients to take on new ones.'

So effective is Knock in medicalising the town that when Dr Parpalaid returns three months later to collect the outstanding payment for the sale of the practice, he finds the local Hôtel de la Clef full of patients. The chambermaid (now nurse assistant) fails to recognise Dr Parpalaid and innocently insults him by adding that she hadn't known there was a doctor in town before Dr Knock. Mousquet is run off his feet with work, and loving it: 'it's not the old cabbage patch life of the old days'. Mr Bernard, the schoolteacher, has moved on to giving illustrated public lectures on the need for perpetual readiness against the menace of the microbe. Public health was a major concern in the France that had lost ten percent of its male population to the Great War: even Louis-Ferdinand Céline—a.k.a. Dr Destouches, urban nihilist and Proust's closest rival for the title of greatest French novelist of the century—did his stint to improve the stock of future generations, touring Brittany in a Rockefeller-funded campaign against tuberculosis in the period in which *Knock* was written, when he would sing, to presumably startled schoolchildren, '*va-t-en, va-t-en microbe!*' to the tune of '*Il pleut, il pleut, bergère*'.

That these campaigns against the unseen menace in the midst of the French population were not without effect can be surmised from the habits of an unquestionably intelligent middle-class family of the period: Simone Weil's biographer David McLellan reports that in the 1910s her entire family (which was a medical one), lived in fear of microbes and went about obsessively washing hands, opening doors with elbows and generally shunning intimate contact.

Knock astounds his predecessor with his figures for the last three months, and not just the consultation rates: he knows the incomes of every household in the canton. But it's not their money he's after, he assures Parpalaid: he has brought people to medicine, he has given their lives a medical meaning. In the long monologue at the end of the play he introduces the pathos of 250 households *où quelqu'un confesse la médecine*, not to mention the climactic prospect of 250 rectal temperatures about to be read simultaneously. He asks Dr Parpalaid to reconsider the view out of the practice window:

> You were contemplating a wild landscape, barely cultivated by human hand. Now I offer it to you impregnated by medicine, fired by the spirit of our subterranean art. When I stood here for the first time, the day after my arrival, I wasn't too proud: I realised my presence didn't count for much. This vast expanse of France had the temerity to spurn me and my coevals. But now I'm as much at ease here as an organist sitting down to play his instrument. In two hundred and fifty of these houses—not all of which are apparent because of the distance and the greenery—there are two hundred and fifty bedrooms where someone's confessing the power of medicine, two hundred and fifty beds where a recumbent body attests that life has a purpose, and—thanks to me—a medical purpose. At night the view is even more beautiful, for then their lights shine out. And almost all these lights are mine. Non-patients sleep in the outer dark. They cease to exist. But patients leave on their night-lights or their lamps. For me, night banishes everything that remains outside medicine, wipes away its irritation and

provocation. Instead of the district we know there is a kind of firmament of which I am the continual creator. And I haven't mentioned the bells. Their first office for all these people is call them to my prescriptions; the bells intone my orders. Think of it: in a few moments, ten o'clock is going to sound, and for all my patients ten o'clock is when they read their rectal temperature for the second time: just think, in a few moments, two hundred and fifty thermometers will be inserted at the same time...

Knock is acting not for his own good, he tells Parpalaid, nor even that of his patients, but in the interests of that third thing: *la médecine*. Parpalaid is struck dumb, bereft of argument; though Knock's claim to be serving higher interests should have alarmed him: here is a physician whose ethics come from Plato not Hippocrates. Without an effective riposte, the conclusion is foregone: soon the old doctor, who has already had to suffer the ignominy of his less than rapturous welcome by the hotel/hospital staff, and who would seem to be the person best armed through his culture and experience to recognise Knock for what he is—an agent of the great Lie—and thereby resist his blandishments, is being invited by his successor for a rest cure himself. Knock's medicalisation of the canton is complete.

Progress has come to Saint-Maurice, so it believes, and it is a collective progress which nobody has the power to resist, not even Dr Parpalaid. A self-contained society forms as the spectator watches; it shares the same hopes and fears, its solidarity is such, even after three months, as to repulse Dr Parpalaid when he comes to collect the remaining payment on his old practice. Whatever fails to fit this world as interpreted by medicine is suppressed or rejected: medicine for the inhabitants of Saint Maurice is now the very content of their lives. They offer Knock a seller's market. He leans on what he is expert at inducing—fear: a contrived dart of panic that can make laughter from spectators sound oddly complicit and uneasy. The inhabitants of St Maurice might be suffering from *maladies imaginaires*, but Knock is a master at the art of reinforcing that particular form of fright. His strategy is simple but effective: he defines the bad, dictates the good. He invokes a cosmic principle, subjecting the horizontal society of supposedly autonomous subjects to the vertical idea—of divinity. Perhaps he is a latter-day Dr Mesmer, a magnetiser who makes the instruments of reason minister to a prospect of salvation, plumbing that part of the mind that is ineducable, a metaphoric but no less fateful *terra incognita* the French psychologist Pierre Janet termed 'the subconscious' five years before Freud.

Hygiene and politics

What gives pause in Romains' brilliant farce is that when it appeared, in the polarised interbellum in which the liberal consensus seemed doomed to disappear and Europe's cultural avant-garde lent its support to new, illiberal forms of modernisation, *Knock* was interpreted as a parable about demagogues who seemed able to mould entire populations to their will. Knock was a type of Great Dictator, the politician with big plans: a few years after the first stage performance of *Knock*, Thomas Mann published his novel *Mario and the Magician* (*Mario und der Zauberer*), the story of a hunchbacked conjurer and 'mind-reader' Cipolla, who plays the audience in the southern Italian resort of Torre di Venere with his hypnotic patter—mixed in with a good deal of patriotic fervour and xenophobia. He tries to persuade a waiter called Mario to kiss him in public; instead Mario shoots him dead. Mann was fascinated by 'primitive mass-democratic funfair vulgarity' and the sometimes dubious figure of the 'artist'. He spent his last years in Switzerland writing a novelistic version of a short story *Confessions of Felix Krull, Confidence Man* (*Bekenntnisse des Hochstaplers Felix Krull*) which had first appeared in book form in the same year as *Knock*, 1922. Felix Krull was a high-society impostor who moved easily across a histrionic frontier between ideology and vaude-ville knavery. That had been the year, too, when Mussolini—'Il Duce'—came to power in Italy.

There are parallels. The more daringly absolute Knock's demands on the Saint-Mauriciens—he even gets the Lady in Black, who exudes 'peasant avarice and constipation', to renounce what is clearly her only real passion in life, *la bouffe*—the more certain they are of his authority to impose such strictures upon them. Their microcosm, even though it is rural, has no socially cohe-sive institution to counteract medicine's explaining power (hence

Knock's interest in Act I in discovering whether the townspeople regularly attend Mass—white or black). Knock lacks any sense of scruple or limit, though he repeatedly claims to be the servant of a higher morality. He plays up to his patients' *amour propre*, while drastically curtailing their freedom. Sacrifices there will have to be. Soon his patients are running after something they already have. Mark Twain noted, with his usual pawky humour, how little of substance is actually offered by health messiahs: 'There are people who strictly deprive themselves of each and every eatable, drinkable and smokeable which has in any way acquired a shady reputation. They pay this price for health. And health is all they get out of it. How strange it is. It is like paying out your whole fortune for a cow that has gone dry.' Or it could be that Knock is in thrall to an impersonal will-to-diagnosis: in the last scene of the play he tells Dr Parpalaid that his 'involuntary diagnosis-making' has become so highly developed he dare not look in the mirror.

Romains must have been familiar with the book *Self-Mastery Through Conscious Auto-Suggestion* (1922) by Emile Coué ('every day, in every way, I grow better and better'), expounder of a muddleheaded belief in the 'science' of self-improvement which enjoyed a massive vogue between the wars, as well as Nietzsche's visionary portrait of the 'great deceivers', salesmen who end up as their own first customers: '*The point of honesty in deception*: In all great deceivers there takes place a remarkable process to which they owe their power. In the very act of deception with all its preparations, the dreadful voice and expression and gestures, amid the whole effective scenario, the *belief in themselves* overcomes them; and it is this belief which then speaks so miraculously, so persuasively, to their audience. [...] For humans believe something to be true if they see others firmly believe in it.' (*Human, All Too Human*, § 52.)

In 1923, Knock's claims to effectiveness were mostly laughable. The farce was still a game. Medicine lacked sufficient prestige for its authority to be recognised as anything like a law of nature, as Simone Weil pointed out in her essay *The Power of Words*. She comments specifically on the power of institutions to 'secrete' abstractions: 'This particular kind of secretion is wonderfully illustrated by Jules Romains' *Knock* with his maxim: "Above the interest of the patient and the interest of the doctor stands the interest of Medicine." It is pure comedy, since the medical profession has not so far secreted such an entity.'

Not so far? Exactly a decade later German doctors were among the most enthusiastic supporters of the social mutations of Hitler's New Republic, servants of a Medicine whose aims were ideological, over and above the interest of individuals. Doctors were feted as warriors in white coats, for National Socialism was nothing else but 'politically applied biology' (Hans Schemm, 1934). The Nazi ethos was actually based on a *sacred* biology, its internal logic consistent with the Nazi belief that the party had been ordained to shape the world's destiny, a destiny which itself would be biological. Science wrote the libretto, Wagner provided the orchestration. Robert Proctor's study of public health policies during that period categorises Nazism as 'a vast hygienic experiment designed to bring about an exclusionist sanitary utopia': paranoia about contamination and pollution wasn't just metaphorical, it served as a spur to concerted attempts at engineering the health of the German population. Studies were launched into environmental hazards, and efforts were made to improve the German diet and reduce alcoholism. Hitler, as everyone knows, was a non-smoking teetotaller. The Nazi example is extreme, but it reveals the thinness of the line between individual liberty and public compulsion: in a sense, public health is medicine's *peccatum originarium*, subverting its proper concern with the individual that has come down from Hippocrates.

But where would we be without public health and decent living conditions? A *Times* editorial of 1854, when medical scientists still believed that infectious diseases were caused by miasma or bad air, thundered against John Snow's attempts to improve the sanitary quality of drinking water by shutting down the communal pump in Broad Street: 'We prefer to take our chance with cholera than be bullied into health.' How many club-members folded up their newspapers, one wonders, and wandered down through Soho to Broad Street, in a London lit by the new gas, in order to test their principles directly at source?

Knock and the future

After the war, Romains' prescience about the great dictators was acknowledged in the breach, though any comfort it might have brought him—vilified in the collaborationist press, witness to the disgrace of France, and deprived of the moral support of his friend Stefan Zweig, who committed suicide in 1942 in Brazil—must have been slight. Cold-war Europe was no longer the continent he had striven to save. He ended his days, in that famous retirement home for distinguished French writers and thinkers, the Académie française.

It was left to Louis Jouvet, in an article published to conclude a conference at the Université des Annales in 1949, to show how well he understood the ambiguous appeal of the play and its eponymous character: 'Twenty-five years ago, in a penetrating act of inspiration, *Knock* revealed the direction a new mentality was going to take. [...] This mentality was Information and its strategies, astounding advances and violent dramatisings; abrupt and terrifying revelations; the invention of new needs, new ways of breakdown; the exalting of fresh anxieties that humankind would feed upon. Jules Romains announced, though we didn't yet know it, the mad-cap mechanisms that were going to rule the world, suggestion and self-suggestion. In *Knock*, like a prophet at the gates, Jules Romains suddenly shone a light on power, the upsurge of guiding concepts (*idées-forces*) and collective theories. Humankind is a machine to make gods and every leader of men a creator of myths. Jules Romains, philosopher, moralist and dramatist, provided an admirable advance warning of the modern and all-encompassing mechanism of cohesion and conviction...'

Romains' play is still read and studied by French schoolchildren, which is cheering. But it seems to have had little effect as critique on the original experimental society: France is now one of the most highly medicalised countries in the world. The post-war period saw the medicalisation of France in the grand style, a process dramatically accelerated by the events of summer 1968. '*Knockisme*' has entered the French language, and is used occasionally in medical anthropology as a descriptive term for popular credulity and gullibility. Yet the play is more than a study of dupery: the Italian philologist Guido Ceronetti noted that all the old satires on medicine and doctors look backwards, over their shoulder;

Knock, on the other hand, steps confidently into the future. It is a play that capitalizes on Marx's idea of tragedy reinstated as farce—except that the farce comes first and the tragedy later. The villain of the piece allows himself a smile just once in the play (or rather the film), while reading the town crier's mind. He has made a discovery, and it isn't medical but mythic. In the great Lie, wrote Hitler, there is always a certain force of credibility. It is the powerful who smile this way: it is a signal of their ironic treatment of social conventions, as if laws existed only for the stupid. Knock has found a way to deflect hubris. By deflecting it from himself, he obliges Nemesis to visit those who take him at his word. Nemesis is user-friendly and not at all dramatic, ladies and gentlemen, for these are modern times—Nemesis is the realisation that desire is both prerational and manufactured to the highest quality standards. Nemesis is the actor acted upon. Just look around. Despite all our best efforts illness refuses to disappear. It takes on new forms; it turns up where nobody left it; it gets invented by the institutions set up by the political and social relations of civilisation itself, which include the medical profession. Then the misfortunes to which doctors owe their livelihood—disease is, at least, a *natural* evil—become ambiguous in hitherto unsuspected ways. People start to visit the doctor not so much because they are ill, but because they are unable to be healthy. Soon doctors start to resemble lawyers, who also owe their livelihood to an evil, but not a natural one. And before we know it, we are opening the door on the world of Knock's higher cynicism: with his right hand he accepts the fee for stilling the devil set loose with his left...

But that left hand has created a community of interests. Knock treats the people of Saint Maurice coldly, like an anthropologist. He simplifies what he says, then repeats himself. Isn't it that people ask to be deceived? Alright, he will deceive them. Order requires domination, and domination requires a lie or two. So he gives their lives a medical meaning. That is: he extends the bounds of the biological, of whose oracles he is the interpreter, so as to make illness not just a bodily phenomenon but an organising principle for the effective administration of society itself: it is, for its adepts, a higher truth. His argument is life, for that is what a doctor defends. His tools are ideals, seduction, fright and—if necessary—the threat of violence. His power is his command of language; in that respect nothing has changed since Molière's day: Knock is as much a storyteller, raconteur, bluffer, salesman and 'habile homme' as Sganarelle, who was a subversive valet and sham doctor. But who's talking sham? Knock gives everyone the fever. Then he inoculates his patients with the one idea: self-preservation, at any cost.

We have to go back to the beginnings of Enlightenment and the twilight of the traditional world from which doctors derive their sacerdotal aura to find out why. The first realisation that the equation 'knowledge is power'—Knock's recipe—could turn in on itself, through the force of imagination, is to be found in the work of one of the wittiest and most clear-sighted philosophers of the period, Georg Christoph Lichtenberg (1742–1799). Around the time of the French Revolution—that historical rupture that changed the role and status of the medical profession for better and worse—he wrote a short but pregnant aphorism. 'Health,' he told his scrapbook, 'is contagious.'

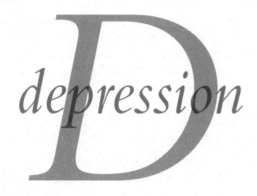

depression

A Conspiracy of Good Intentions

PROZAC AND ITS IMITATORS

Prozac®, as Carl Elliott writes in the introduction to *Prozac as a Way of Life*, may have begun life as a brand name for the active ingredient fluoxetine, but it is now a descriptive epithet for the entire family of selective serotonin reuptake inhibitor drugs (SSRIs), and, by extension, a lifestyle. When people say Prozac they may well be talking about something else, for Prozac has been so successful since being launched on the market that it has reared offspring: Paxil® (paroxetine), Luvox® (fluvoxetine), Zoloft® (sertraline), Effexor® (venlefaxine) and Celexa® (citalopram). And the number of disorders these drugs are licensed to treat has broadened well beyond depression to include conditions all but invisible until the 1990s: social phobia, panic disorders, eating disorders, post-traumatic stress disorder and sexual compulsions. When Eli Lilly's patent for Prozac expired in 2001 it was marketed under a different name, Sarafem®, as a treatment for 'premenstrual dysphoric disorder'. The bottom line would seem to be: if you want to sell drugs, sell the disorder first.

Prozac as a Way of Life, eleven essays by different hands, is an unusually literate attempt to take the measure of the world that made Prozac and its corollary: the world that Prozac is making. Prozac has been with us long enough now for it to have gone the way of all drugs: first its acclamation as the universal panacea, then media boosting, followed by the slow emergence of doubt, media quickening of doubt, and finally the backlash (we are currently between stages four and five).

If Prozac has the ability to alter feelings and actions, reshaping what we call empathy, the bonds of mutuality between individuals, then it has the ability to reshape the fabric of life itself. What can be said about the place in society that the SSRIs have come to occupy? Does it bear any resemblance to the situation in the 1960s, when Valium®—'Mother's little helper', as the Rolling Stones mocked it—was prescribed in large quantities to help women endure what Erik Parens in this book calls 'patently unjust social arrangements and attitudes'? Can Prozac truly be a liberating drug, as many of its supporters claim, when its use increases dependency, if only the minimal dependency of patient on industry (not to mention medical profession)? If the bulimic consumption of antidepressants betrays an essential *lack*, what is it people are missing? Or do antidepressants in some as yet poorly understood way 'recruit' those patients who are likely to respond to them? And then there is the libertarian twister: if every culture has its licit psychoactive substances, from betel nuts and kava to alcohol and nicotine, why should the medical profession be the sole guardian of access to SSRIs?

Depression is our contemporary diagnostic black hole. Consider the statistics: from being a rare diagnosis (affecting perhaps fifty people per million) in 1957, when the first antidepressant was discovered, by 1970 the number of depressed persons was estimated by the psychiatrist Heinz Lehmann to be one hundred million worldwide. The Swiss pharmaceutical company Geigy actually decided not to develop imipramine in the 1950s on the grounds that the market was too sluggish to provide a return on investment. In the 1980s, the number of depressed patients on treatment in France alone increased by one million. In the USA prescriptions for SSRIs increased by 20.9% in a single year (1999–2000). According to the World Health Organization, depression and cardiovascular disease are set to be the two major public health problems of the third millennium: the prevalence of depression in the world's population is three percent. Prozac has excited the philosophers and ethicists in a way that imipramine did not (as exemplified by Peter Kramer's best-seller *Listening to Prozac*).

This suggests we are facing a phenomenon not just of medical or sociological importance, but a radical anthropological change, and a mutation in the way we think about ourselves. You can't argue with success, but it looks as if we should, and in fairly sober words. Calling Prozac 'Zen medicine', as Susan Squier does, merely ushers us all the more completely into a kind of semantic overload while obscuring the material origin of signs in the bodies whose productive activities provide the continuity that might help us, as *subjects*, to avoid full-scale medicalisation.

The key essay in the collection is David Healy's conference paper 'Good Science or Good Business?' It was publication of this account of a possible link between Prozac and suicide in the *Hastings Center Report* which led, controversially, to the rescinding of Healy's appointment to a post in Toronto. (The event brought into question the very impartiality of bioethicists in the United States, all too many of them being in receipt of funding from corporate bodies.) Healy outlines how the regulatory response to the thalidomide disaster in the 1960s—in which thousands of infants were born with congenital defects after the German company Grünenthal marketed it as an over-the-counter remedy for nausea in pregnant women—gave rise to the 'disease states' that are now essential to secure FDA approval for any new medication. For years the pharmaceutical industry has been putting vast resources into gathering and disseminating information to influence treatment lobbies and the manner in which doctors prescribe. Nearly all university research has some involvement with the industry, which may also be funding some patient support groups (Eli Lilly funds the National Alliance for the Mentally Ill in the USA, for instance). Experts often rotate between sectors, so that a government adviser may previously have worked for the private sector, or directly for the industry itself. As Laurence Kirmayer says in his article on the quite different cultural experience with Prozac in Japan, 'professional autonomy rides the tail of marketing'. The advertising budget for Prozac actually exceeds the already bloated budget for Nike running shoes. Even those last bastions of objectivity in science, the medical journals, are not protected from the pressures and forces of the market: Richard Horton, editor of *The Lancet*, has written that '[they] have devolved into information-laundering operations for the pharmaceutical industry'. Studies have shown that doctors tend rather complacently to underestimate the hold the pharmaceutical industry has over them. Furthermore, most practitioners are naïve realists—which is to say that they treat their patients in good faith, assuming them to be genuinely ill—and patients present with genuine symptoms (which must be genuine since they've just been ticked off on the symptom list). Nobody appears to be trying to put one over on anyone else. Yet Healy suggests that Prozac is *less* likely to 'work' when its effects are evaluated using patient-based, non-specific quality of life arguments rather than clinician-based rating scales (as would be adopted in a single- or double-blind trial). We also know that approximately one third of all depressed patients respond positively to a placebo, though this finding is manifestly of little interest to the pharmaceutical companies.

So what order of phenomenon are we dealing with? Can it be that modern psychiatry is based on something like a category error brought about by the triumph of the biological model of disease in a society that values individual initiative above all else while blinding itself to those aspects of mind that reveal it as something *shared*?

This is the contention defended by Thomas Szasz, who in his defence of classic liberalism has repeatedly and paradoxically drawn attention to the fact that mental disorders are above all *metaphorical* illnesses. 'What people nowadays call mental illness, especially in a legal context, is not a fact, but a strategy; not a condition, but a policy.' If depression did have an infectious cause, the figures quoted above would be alarming though not altogether surprising: in the lack of anything like a necessary and sufficient cause, the only statement we can confidently venture is the circular argument that depression is the state of mind which antidepressants are able to act upon.

Wherein lies the 'contagion' then? One possibility we are forced to consider is that the mind is a rather susceptible receiver of electromagnetically-mediated image-driven consciousness rather than the producer of the rare and difficult predicative knowledge (of the form 'A is B') that is a feature of genuine science. Wasn't that precisely why Plato sought to condemn the scandal of mimetic poetry and myth in Book 10 of *The Republic*? Isn't that the whole force of the religious critique of idolatry?

Prozac as a Way of Life lacks the historical long view. One thread that ought to be running through it is the (American) search for the authentic self, although those who chase the drug bandwagon are manifestly slaves to a conformism that makes the whole idea of authenticity look like a bad joke. The body-blow dealt by the Vietnam War to the onward march of the American dream surely deserves consideration: the rise of post-traumatic stress disorder (PTSD) offers an intriguing parallel with that of depression. This label gave war veterans a kind of moral legitimacy, and guaranteed them a disability pension. The Victorian imperial personality—disciplined, rule-observant, respectful of authority and fairly sure of its entitlements—survived until the 1950s, and perhaps a few years longer in Britain (which had its 1968 revolt twenty years after everyone else); the new individual of the age of bounty is caught on the rack between what is permitted and what is possible. Choice is the mantra, although the 'choices' increasingly look stage-managed. One aspect of the old-fashioned bourgeois life that is easily overlooked is its dignity, but it was a dignity that insisted on making distinctions between realms of experience in order to wring order from a truculent and harsh reality. The cost of contemporary liberation from socially ascribed rituals, practices and even family links is a kind of free-floating anxiety. For the one condition that describes our life is its *optionality*. Many commentators bemoan 'the loss of values' in contemporary society, the fact that people don't 'believe' in anything any more. Who's kidding whom! Every aspect of contemporary life is bogged down in morality, especially the morality of doing your own thing while looking over your shoulder to make sure that next door is doing hers too. It would seem that the desire to authenticate the stirrings of the will is essentially a form of Puritanism. Despite the rhetoric of liberation, we are still within the tight little orbits of Calvinist self-justification.

In the old Soviet Union, people who criticised the system were sent to psychiatric institutions for 'correction' or 're-education':

the putative citizens of the expertocracies of the twenty-first century, on the other hand, are likely to be so well-trained that if they feel a phobic phase coming on (i.e. an urge to criticise the radiant society erecting itself around them) they won't commit themselves to an institution—they'll just self-medicate. Well, that was what radical critics used to promote in the 1960s when almost every commodity in Western culture pretended to offer some kind of psychedelic experience; but it is salutary to remember too what Orwell wrote about Swift's Houyhnynms: 'They had reached, in fact, the highest stage of totalitarian organisation when conformity has become so general that there is no need for a police force.'

Odd as it sounds, the more private and uniform (that is, the more autistic) it becomes, the more the techno-pantheistic self is forced to model its behaviour on others. It is a kind of liberated false consciousness bound by the same logic as Chesterton's brilliant quip in *Heretics* about 'the globetrotter living in a smaller world than the peasant'. That is why the latest generation of psychoactive drugs is almost certainly, to borrow a phrase from Karl Kraus, the disorder to which it purports to be the cure.

In the ever more complex and impersonal division of labour in modern society, depression might be seen as a kind of decompression of the individual working part, clueless as to its place in the meaningful whole: this decompression is one of the inevitable 'transaction costs' incurred by the complexity of the system, and one which can be cynically accepted provided the system continues to be ever more productive. Antidepressants will therefore intensify the problems they appear to resolve (and that goes for other 'pharmacratic' developments such as Ritalin® and the so-called 'attention deficit hyperactivity syndrome'). Kraus' aphorism restates our syllogism: supply leads demand, rhetoric prompts discourse, outcome trumps genesis. It suggests that in our society, which posits agency in terms of the individual actor *making* decisions, it is actually the robust, impersonal and pragmatic empiricism of the great social experiment embarked upon several centuries ago (look: no Experimenter!) that now carries the day: last things come first. Reality has become the endless speculative fairground described by Leibniz even though we still don't understand anything very much at all about the relationship between consciousness and its physical embodiment: who we are, where we are or even *when* we are.

Prozac as a Way of Life provides some helpful approaches towards an understanding of how depression has become an epidemic. As Robert Burton suggested, in his solid and (I presume) widely unread classic of the English language *The Anatomy of Melancholy*, published in 1621 when the humoral theory of disease was about to be overtaken by the new vocabulary of contagion and commodities, one of the symptoms of melancholia is not to know its cause. That cause may be civic in origin, not just a sickness of the soul.

Mention of Burton reminds me that I was once moved, in what I thought was a refreshing turn of honesty but probably came over as a brutal quirk of exasperation, to suggest to one of my patients at the end of a long and not very productive consultation, 'You're not depressed, you're unhappy, and only you know why.' My patient looked shocked: how should *I* know what is wrong with me when *he* refuses to say? That was the last I saw of her.

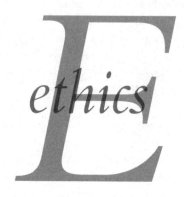

Insomnia
(in the Bed of Being)

The philosophy of non-sleep

Vladimir Nabokov wrote that the world's population divides into two categories: those who sleep peacefully at night, and those who sleep badly. He himself was a notorious insomniac: he was afraid of the night, which he called a 'giant'.

E. M. Cioran, the Romanian desperado who became a distinguished French writer, was of the same opinion. 'Human beings,' he wrote in *History and Utopia*, 'are divided into *sleepers* and *wakers*, two specimens of being forever distinct from the other, with nothing but their physical aspect in common.' This, he thought, was enough to account for a person's 'extravagances', although what he had in mind was surely his own writing style. In 1982, he wrote: 'It's not so overwhelmingly bad to have suffered from insomnia in youth, because it opens your eyes. It's an extremely painful experience, a catastrophe. But it makes you understand things which other people can't: insomnia puts you outside the living, outside humanity. You're excluded. [...] What is insomnia? At eight o'clock in the morning you're exactly where you were at eight in the evening! There's no progress. There's only this immense night around you. And life is only possible through the discontinuity which sleep gives it. The disappearance of sleep creates a sort of dreary continuity.'

Cioran is clearly an ungrateful descendant of the two little children in Adalbert Stifter's famous Christmas story *Rock Crystal* who err in a snow-storm on their way home to their alpine village in the next valley and end up on a glacier shelf. These 'tiny moving dots among the formidable masses' seek shelter in a bedrock cave. Safe at least from the world-obliterating blizzard outside, they dare not close their eyes for fear of freezing and becoming part of the stone and ice around them. They sit in the emptiness of the hours to come as well as in the surrounding immensity. It is not just the black coffee extract they drink that saves them from the sleep 'whose seductiveness invariably gets the better of reason': something of the grandeur of Nature itself wakens in them a resistance and wakefulness strong enough to withstand its most hostile forces. The brother and sister in Stifter's story have each other for company; Cioran had only himself. (Or so he liked to pretend: his companion Simone Boué provided for his bodily needs for the decades in which he was reputed not to have slept, and even edited his notebooks, but doesn't appear once in his voluminous writings.)

Cioran wasn't suffering from simple sleep loss. He had forfeited the right to sleep, possibly because he knew too intimately the chaos of history and his own role in it. His insomnia was a double privation. In the several interviews he gave late in life he often referred to the boyhood experience of having to leave his native village of Rǎşinari for the considerably larger city of Sibiu (also known, like everywhere else in that part of the world, by another two names: as Nagyszeben and Hermannstadt). The Transylvanian capital was then a part of the Austro-Hungarian Empire and for centuries had been considered one of the outposts of Europe. Little Emil cried, inconsolably, all the way to town.

Cioran's sleeplessness in the dead time was a stylised form of the apprehensiveness expressed by another writer adopted by the French—the philosopher Emmanuel Levinas. He had an oceanic phrase for it: 'insomnia in the bed of being'.

'A kind of closing of the eyes'

Writers, it might be thought, are typical wakers: their imaginative life is always at a tangent to ordinary social life, and not only for economic reasons. Literature is often a pursuit in the counterglow: only night offers the quietness in which a person can school himself to work in the absence of those who have long since turned in.

Franz Kafka complained much about sleeplessness as he wrote into the small hours. He felt like a sentry on cosmic guard duty at the boundary of consciousness, a soldier on the Great Wall between belief and unbelief, fearful he might lose his life should he fall asleep. Guarding his appended body was what he was there to do, to neutralise all threats to it and secure its workings. Yet with so much effort being given over to staying awake in order to keep watch over his organs, sleep was bound to seem enticing. 'There is, in Kafka,' observed Elias Canetti, 'a sort of sleep-worship; he regards sleep as a panacea.'

In fact Kafka, as even his most admiring critics concede, could be nearly autistic in his detachment from social reality. Kafka's attention to language neglected the etymology of the word: to be attentive (from the Latin verb *attendere*) means to stretch out towards, to bend to another person's presence. Writing is a solitary activity; insomnia had broken the tacit social contract with the family. Avoiding sleep offered him a sense of hyperarousal: that was when he felt most able to write. Hyperarousal was insomnia's vertigo. 'Only *in this way* can writing be done', he told his diary in September 1913, having spent all eight hours of the night writing his first successful story *The Judgement*, his legs so stiff in the morning he could hardly dislodge them from beneath the table. He had been making literature out of an unclaimed portion of universal sleep.

Yet chronic sleep deprivation has its dangers, as Kafka well knew—as well as posing problems for a man who was a civil servant and factory owner in his daytime hours. 'There are moments at the office while talking or dictating', he told his correspondent Grete Bloch in 1914, 'when I am more truly asleep than when I sleep.'

Although he wasn't past taking a tablet or two of Benzedrine to help him meet the deadline on a commissioned piece, W. H. Auden was no night-owl, and even distrusted writing that smelled of the candle—what his classical model Horace might have called 'lucubrationes'. Auden wrote in *Hic et Ille*, 'if you really wish to destroy a person […] the surest method is not physical torture, in the strict sense, but simply to keep him awake, i.e., in an existential relation to life without intermission.' Seeing in the dark is one thing; seeing the dark another. Try to dispense with sleep several nights in a row and you are likely to end up institutionalised, and in an appalling state of psychotic dispersion.

Auden was an avid reader of *Scientific American*: he would have read about the sleep deprivation experiments of the 1950s, the findings of which were avidly adopted by intelligence services as a way of obtaining cooperative detainees. Sleep deprivation was a torture method. Nowadays we seem to be happy to do the torturing by ourselves, on ourselves. Doctors report a vast increase in restlessness, irritability and inability to cope at work, school or with others, not least in children. These cases of transient insomnia aren't army-sanctioned experiments in existential tension; they're the result of people spending too much time interfacing with their gadgets. We've gone into voluntary self-detention. In fact, only a very few people have a genuinely low need for sleep (and still feel rested during the day): they mostly end up as politicians, captains of industry and chefs. The rest of us become sleep debtors.

Friedrich Nietzsche, a sensitive diviner of new cultural trends, thought there was something pathological about the nineteenth-century's obsession with the past. He likened it to a kind of insomnia. Sleep is a desirable state; it allows humans not so much to repose as to *forget*. In his eyes the great reading public, so eager to recuperate its own history, was about to have a collective breakdown through lack of sleep—a lack of sleep so comprehensive, at any rate, as to induce forgetfulness. He had one or two experiences of going without sleep himself, until his mind gave out. Nietzsche couldn't have anticipated that Sigmund Freud, who owed so much to his writings, was about to extend civilisational memory all the way back to the clay tablets of Uruk, in Mesopotamia: Freud was to become one of the great modern dream-readers. It was perhaps only there—after anamnestic descent to the Land of the Great Rivers—that memory could truly go to sleep. James Joyce, too, associated the Tower of Babel with sleep, perhaps in consideration of that great line from *The Epic of Gilgamesh*, written in cuneiform before almost anything else in history but first read with new eyes just over a century ago: 'Sleep, which spills over people, overcame him.'

Gilgamesh's epic might be over four thousand years old but it was our great-grandparents who read it with true discernment. Rainer Maria Rilke was one of the first writers to appreciate its originality after it was deciphered at the end of the nineteenth century: in 1916 he wrote, '*Gilgamesh* is stupendous! I [...] consider it to be among the greatest things that can happen to a person.' Elias Canetti was even more fulsome: the story of Gilgamesh had a crucial impact on his intimate life 'such as nothing else in the world'.

Narcolepsy and wakefulness

Sleep, insomnia, oneiric states: they were all in the air of the early twentieth century. Nicolas Vaschede, a professional physiologist, confirmed in 1914 that sleep isn't just the absence of being awake, but an active biological process. All animals seem to do it; some standing erect (horses), others on the wing (migrating birds). Herbivores sleep less than carnivores, having much to fear from the stealth of the latter. Sleep certainly has its natural archaeology, but it took until the 1950s for scientists to understand fully its dynamic, oscillating nature, and the importance of what is called rapid eye movement (REM) sleep, especially in infant life. Even then biology may well be inflected by cultural practices: people in traditional societies (who go to bed when the light fades) often get up in the middle of the night to engage for a while in social activities, and our immediate ancestors often rose to pray for an hour or two before reclining again on the pillow. The odd thing is: we don't understand *why* we sleep. William Dement, the American scientist who mapped sleep architecture in more detail than almost anyone else, wrote at the end of his career that 'the only reason we need to sleep that is really, really solid, is that we get sleepy'—and that is less a reason than a precondition.

Sleep begets sleep. Or rather, going to sleep is a strange ritual in which the body pretends to be sleeping in order for the mind to become dormant.

Vaschede's contemporary, that amateur literary scientist Marcel Proust, assures us in his contemporaneous giant work of extended physiology *À la Recherche du Temps Perdu*, that sleep is 'the most potent of hypnotics'. No kidding! The opening pages of his famous work are certainly contagious; for years I could never advance further into his novel because, reading it in bed, I found the overture, which describes his character Swann talking about his sleep experiences, sent me into the thing itself. And once you're in it, the labyrinth of sleep ignores the law of time: Swann's attempt to wake up 'consisted above all in an attempt to introduce the obscure, undefined block of sleep that [he] had just been living into the framework of time.' Somehow, the living daylights resume. Never have those hypnopompic moments of wakening 'behind a vestment of oblivion' (as the frontal lobe returns us to the world in the first few minutes of awakening) been more lyrically evoked: Proust has a fantastic word for the illusion of hearing bells in his dreams: he calls them 'aeroliths'. (There have been times when I thought I was hearing the bells of Combray too, but their peal always turned out to be the chime of my old-fashioned alarm clock.)

Proust was unfamiliar with rural Ireland though. Flann O'Brien made much of his country's soporific culture and populated his novels with narcoleptic characters ready at a moment's notice to fall asleep, even in public. His savant hero De Selby in *The Third Policeman* muses to himself that sleep is 'an immeasurable boon', not least on account of his own habit of nodding off opportunely. 'Several times I had gone asleep when my brain could no longer bear the situation it was faced with.' If only it were that easy! His assumption suggests a country where the characters are neither quite alive nor quite dead, although the phenomenon known as a microsleep, in which the mind momentarily disengages with the waking world, is by no means uncommon or restricted to Ireland.

It is true that a degree of disengagement or even a state of torpor may be necessary to assimilate some experiences. Walter Benjamin, in his famous essay on storytelling, suggested that the repose of a sleeping person finds an analogy in boredom, 'the apogee of mental relaxation', which he thought was becoming an ever less common feature of modern life. In this state of self-forgetful reverie, we are receptive in depth. 'Boredom is the dream bird that hatches the egg of experience', he suggested in his famous essay *The Storyteller*. 'A rustling in the leaves drives it away.'

Flann O'Brien's sleep-blanketed Ireland could never know the existential pangs of Cioran's world. Yet a kind of tonelessness adheres to them both. *Une nuit blanche*—the French term for a sleepless night—is the most exquisite torture, according to Cioran. 'You emerge in fragments, stupid, absent-minded, without recollections or forebodings, and without even knowing who you are. And it's then that the day appears useless, the light pernicious, and even more oppressive than the dark.' (Cioran eventually developed Alzheimer's disease, and there is some evidence to suggest that sleep deprivation may be implicated in its onset.)

The physiologists, professional and amateur, are right: we have an intrinsic biological drive to sleep. Sleep benefits mind and body, and consolidates memories. It might be seductive to have the freedom to work, eat or travel as and when we want, but our bodies have another agenda: under the coordination of a part of the brain called the suprachiasmatic nucleus, the organs of the body actually follow slightly different physiological rhythms. There are even special light receptors in the eye that are uniquely responsive to the blue light of dusk and serve to recalibrate our circadian system: visually blind people are still able to respond to the wax and wane of the cosmos. It is only those who lack ocular bulbs—for whatever reason—who are truly blind.

Subjugating the night, in the manner recommended by so many writers—existential heroes in their own version of the Grimms' story about the boy who set out to discover fear—might seem a victory for culture over biology, but biology is far older than the lights of civilisation, and it is surely an illusion to imagine that we can gain a fuller life by remastering the internal order we share with other living creatures. Nonetheless, the search is on. A recent article announcing the search for a 'cure' for sleep comments: 'Just as the birth control pill uncoupled sex from reproduction, designer stimulants seems poised to remove us yet further from the archaic requirements of the animal kingdom.' Whether they know it or not, wakers who celebrate 'enhancement' (or '150% life') are also cheerleaders for the absolute rule and consumptive tyranny of a 24/7 society.

Sleep is the charity of being alive, much in the same way as forgetting allows us to reconstitute things—even at the risk of repeating ourselves in the most dim-witted, imprudent, injudicious ways. Sleep is where readers are to be found, among aeroliths and sundogs and lucid floaters. There is kind of expansiveness in being a sleeper too. Homer knew that: in his epic poems sleep is a sacred gift. 'For mortals cannot go forever sleepless', Penelope tells the returning Odysseus.

Being permanently awake under modern artificial light might just be a way of withdrawing from the complexity of human life, not least its ethical complexity. Sleep ought to foreshorten time, and restore us, refreshed and purified, to the clarity of a new day. Proust's thesis was that for most of our lives we are asleep to our own true natures, and only waken in the instant we recognise ourselves for what we are. Then, for the length of a lightning flash, our being grasps 'what it normally never apprehends, namely, a fragment of time in its pure state.'

Ethics in the dark

Insomnia in the bed of being: the phrase is a distant reverberation of the first flare of consciousness in the Land of the Two Rivers, some five thousand years ago. As another ancient dream-book has it, the world began with the interruption of a sleep. So what on earth has happened to us, given that most of our working days culminate in a few weary hours staring at indiscreet images on what James Joyce, always alive to the significance of new inventions, called 'the bairdboard bombardment screen'? Surely it is better to say, with the Italian writer Erri de Luca, who gets up each morning at 5 o'clock in order to study the Scriptures in the original Hebrew: 'These pages are not the fruit of insomnia, but of awakenings.' That is the rejuvenating first sentence of his novel *First Light*. He discovered the Bible while working as a jobber on building sites in Paris in the 1980s, and even now, long after he has abandoned hard manual work, still reads it, not as a believer or even a mystic without God, but as somebody who can't get over his surprise every morning at being alive. The only proof of existence is wakefulness. But that doesn't mean reality comes to us spontaneously.

In the Mesopotamian epic, Gilgamesh doesn't want sleep to pour over him. His panic-stricken encounter with death is what the Czech philosopher Jan Patočka called a 'shaking': he moves from the vegetative life of prehistory into the unpredictable and problematic. He becomes *conscious*, and consciousness is like the sky: it is no sheltering vault. Yet consciousness isn't his final self-hood. Gilgamesh is shaken again when his friend Enkidu dies. Fearful of dying himself, he goes on a quest to find Utnapishtim ('the Faraway') and his wife, the only humans to have been granted immortality by the gods after having first (like the biblical Noah) survived the Great Flood. Reaching the island at the end of the world where they live, Gilgamesh discovers that if he wishes to be immortal, he must show he is suited to it: he must stay awake for six days and seven nights.

In spite of all his precautions, he falls asleep. Being immortal clearly isn't worth the candle: nobody wants to experience eternity as a dreary, endless continuity. When he wakens again, Gilgamesh is aghast at his failure to withstand the test. But on his disconsolate return to Uruk, the city he built, he discovers that he is going to enjoy a form of immortality—only it's not going to be the kind he was expecting: he will be remembered as the first civic hero. He is the first builder of city walls, as well of those more abstract partitions that mark out historical eras, political jurisdictions and even the frontiers of finite human lives.

Emmanuel Levinas' philosophy gives priority to the existence of others, their mere presence in the world making demands upon us that are prior to the constitution of the self. Ethics trumps metaphysics. 'It's strange to think', says Eluned Summers-Bremner, author of *Insomnia: A Cultural History*, 'that we might most truthfully enact our belonging to the human community by the act of falling into unconsciousness, the place in which we imagine others to be blissfully dwelling.'

If you find that notion hard to accept then you're almost certainly doing time as an insomniac. Alone, under a cone of light, in the dark.

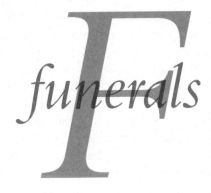

An American Book of the Dead

LIFE STUDIES FROM THE DISMAL TRADE

About 100,000 years ago the fossil record shows our very distant ancestors started tucking their dead under the topsoil. Over a somewhat shorter timescale, but long enough to identify the four horsemen as Stroke, Coronary Occlusion, Alzheimer's and the Big C, Lynch & Sons have kept the tradition going, the American way. The Milford, Michigan end of things is handled by Thomas Lynch, undertaker and poet (*Grimalkin and Other Poems*, 1995). He does the works—embalming, casketing, flower-arranging. If he hasn't got the box your dear departed would have wanted, his brother Tim, working in the next town, can probably supply it. High-temperature exothermic redox combustion can be arranged too, for those few Americans who insist on the somewhat cheaper method of disposal preferred by more than seventy percent of the British population, though few apparently do. The American funeral industry seems to be quite happy to keep things the way they are, embalming and interment and grave maintenance being the last opportunity to fleece the consumer.

Lynch has strong views about why embalming is part of the American way of death, much as he has mordant and occasionally proprietorial views about why we shirk our own undertakings. Some people might find it quite piquant to have flayed cows' heads in formalin looming over them—courtesy of Damien Hirst—while they eat in Soho restaurants, but it would be hard to deny that while death as a shared and communal event is pretty much the distracted reality of late-twentieth century consciousness it has never been more *subjectively* oppressive. Necro-kitsch is one name for what takes its place, and I dare say it won't take very long to find its intellectual equivalent in academic social science curricula. Sure, we talk things to death, and just about every child, it seems, has witnessed thousands of formatted 'TV deaths', but there is no escaping the sense that the symbolic weight of this, after all, most dependable event, has been separated from common life and encysted in individual fears. Perhaps the late Dr Freud might have found it solid confirmation of his Eros and Thanatos equation, obscenity being a more literal-minded word that it used to be.

Indeed, if humankind can be roughly divided, as the Czech poet and immunologist Miroslav Holub has suggested, into those who go hunting and those who clear up the mess afterwards, then undertakers evidently don't have much time to be Hemingways. Thomas Lynch writes about himself as one of the 'dismal traders, funeral types [...] who dress in black, and work the weekends and the holidays, who line the cars and lay the bodies out, who rise and go out in the dark when someone dies and someone calls for help.' Having cleared up a few messes and signed passports for the ultimate journey myself, I was curious to see how things looked from the other end of the table, though I should add that medical qualifications are no prerequisite for reading this book: Lynch has a few telling comments to make about that other Michigan resident, the man who was described in last year's *British Medical Journal* as a 'medical hero'. Dr Jack Kevorkian has now, at the latest body count, had a hand in twenty-eight 'physician-assisted suicides'. Lynch bristles at the oxymoronic notion of anyone being *assisted* 'in [their] one and only suicide' and dubs Kevorkian's idiosyncratic interpretations of a pathologist's duties 'kevorking'. Here he touches on an important argument about a physician's duties to a suffering patient, and asks the perfectly legitimate question: 'Is it possible to assist the ones we love with their dying instead of assisting with their killing?' A retired pathologist on a mission with a self-styled 'Thanatron' in the boot of his car is somehow a very American response to the challenges of providing decent palliative care.

As such observations would suggest, Lynch is neither deaf to the zeitgeist nor a lugubrious *croque-mort*. He comes across as a man of deep feeling and humanity with a keen sense of his Irish Catholic roots. And why shouldn't he be guild-proud, a stickler for detail? Undertaking is a job which requires decorum and decency, a sound grasp of the difference between what happens and what matters, and hangs on a uncommon ability to give form to the messiness of emotions. For a poet, it is nearly native habitat. Lynch tells of an Episcopalian deacon deservedly receiving a verbal cuff from the mother of a newly deceased teenage girl he had been attempting to free from durance with the empty vessel of the professional grief-counsellor—"'I'll tell you when *it's* 'just a shell'", the woman said, "for now and until I tell you otherwise, *she's* my daughter.'" On that scale of delicacy, good undertakers are probably as rare as good poets; Lynch actually steals a couple of recollections of poet-friends into his book, notably of the hypochondriac Matthew Sweeney, 'whose headaches are all brain tumours, his fevers meningitis, his hangovers all peptic ulcers or diverticulitis'. Sweeney comes in for some companionable ribbing for having no sense of what might be beyond 'reasonable doubt': implied criticism, no doubt, but preferable to the ingratiating tone of the praise heaped elsewhere on Lynch's editor Robin Robertson. That minor lapse occurs in an otherwise nicely judged essay called Words Made Flesh, which gives us a fairly close look at Lynch himself (hiding behind the name 'Henry Nugent'), struggling through alcoholism, a marriage breakup and the attendant loneliness. Generally, Lynch is very astute at avoiding the confessional or even flaunting his expertise in what might be called the taxonomy of decay or the more bizarre paraphernalia of his trade.

If undertaking is a calling at 5 AM, it is also a business, and Lynch has a damper for the 'News Hound' at the local television station, whose 'scoop', defying any kind of business sense, is that Lynch & Sons have been selling their caskets for more than they paid for them: Lynch reckons his profit margin is about five percent, which doesn't seem much in a job with such terrible hours. It therefore comes as no surprise that he should remain unperturbed by Jessica Mitford's revelations in *The American Way of Death* or Evelyn Waugh's *The Loved One*, and in what is at once the funniest and harshest essay in the book he sends up the 'What Folks Want in a Casket' approach with a whimsical vision of golf courses doubling as crematoria: 'the combination of golf and good grieving seems a natural, each divisible by the requirement for large tracts of green grass, a concentration on holes, and the need for a someone to carry the bags—caddies or pallbearers'. The same piece contains a rawly moving account of a fellow undertaker working for eighteen hours at no extra pay to reconstruct the staved-in face and skull of a murder victim so that her mother can grieve over her daughter's recognisable remains. '"Barbaric" is what Jessica Mitford called this "fussing over the dead body". I say the monster with the baseball bat was barbaric.' Lynch's comeback seems misplaced; Mitford was targetting corporate takeovers of independent firms like Lynch & Sons, companies such as Service Corporation International with their shareholders and annual report: 'S.C.I. experienced the most dynamic year in its history in 1994, reaching new milestones in revenues and net incomes while establishing a solid presence in the European funeral industry.' (I quote from a March 1997 edition of *Vanity Fair* kindly left by an American patient in my waiting room.)

Recognising ourselves among small acts of kindness, and recognising what is beyond any kindness, might be what this book is urging us towards. Thomas Lynch recognises himself in 'the cardiac blue' of his father—the undertaker overtaken—who had arranged with his sons that they would embalm him when he died, the fearful man whose characteristic first thought in younger life had been to ban his kids from doing the usual things children do because he 'had just buried someone doing the very thing'. Lynch recognises his fellow townspeople by telling them back their own life stories as he prepares them for burial, remembering convivial occasions disrupted by the mixture of fright and curiosity that the profession of making a living from the dead provokes. Vindicating Gladstone's adage, he writes, 'the meaning of life is connected, inextricably, to the meaning of death; that mourning is a romance in reverse, and if you love you grieve and there are no exceptions—only those who do it well and those who don't. And if death is regarded as an embarrassment or an inconvenience, if the dead are regarded as a nuisance from whom we wreak a hurried riddance, then life and the living are in for like treatment: McFunerals, McFamilies, McMarriage, McValues.'

'One so seldom learns the end of things in life', wrote Henry Green in one of the sad little tales in his book of collected short writings, *Surviving*. Given that he has been privy, time and again, to the only end of things, Thomas Lynch's book is almost a miracle of feeling, tact and good sense, a remarkable and unbookish study of all the implications of the word 'undertaking'. Lynch has, in a sense, reclaimed the innocent belief he had of it when he was a child: that his father's job literally involved taking the dead underground. His book is a small classic on the most universal subject, and why the care we give to those who are past caring ultimately reflects how we look to ourselves, alive and civilised. It is a long time indeed since anyone dared write an *ars moriendi*.

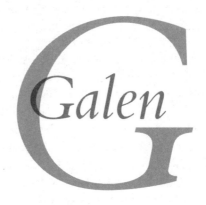

Galen

Crise de Foie

FRENCH MEDICINE AND THE LIVER

FOI (f): (Lat. fides 'bond, engagement') *A belief not founded on rational principles.*

FOIE (m): (Lat. ficatum 'goose liver fattened with figs'): *Organ contained in the abdomen, an extension of the digestive tube, which secretes bile and carries out a number of functions in carbohydrate, lipid and protein metabolism.*

– Petit Larrousse illustré

Until the twentieth-century the history of making a living out of other people's bad days wasn't an edifying one. For close on twenty-two hundred years people thought disease came about if their blood, yellow bile, black bile and what can only be described as slime were not in harmony. The cure was often worse than the disease, yet for all those centuries before the dawn of Incredible Progress doctors never seemed to go out of business.

Now that medicine seems to be limited only by its means, perhaps it's the vestigial memory of quackery, barber-shops and that odd business with leeches that makes the profession unwilling to admit there are things about the body which leave its observer, if not its tenant, nonplussed. And even though scalpels aren't much of a weapon compared to scythes, doctors now think of themselves, with the blessing of society at large, as progressive people at the cutting edge of the possible; that's surely why they get hot under the collar when such nonplussing suggests there is less science in medicine than generally supposed. Particularly if this insight comes from the patient, who may expect his physician to be a soothsayer, prophet and salesman for eternal hope, not just someone insisting that if the one-eyed lead the blind we'll somehow get there.

When I started up my own practice in Strasbourg, where many of my patients speak in strange tongues (twenty-two different nationalities I once worked out), I suffered such a double embarrassment; not merely one over commonplace terms, but also over the kind of bodily reality those terms expressed.

The embarrassment was due to the fact that I didn't know what a *crise de foie* was or how to deal with it. In all my time in medicine, from the mother-country to several of its English speaking daughters, I'd never come across an hepatic storm, an acute liver, bile acid build-up (BABU) or anything else resembling this liverish state of being. Even my own sister, who wrote her PhD thesis on one of the major detoxification pathways in the liver, the cytochrome P450 system, had never heard of it. Something rare like acute intermittent porphyria, about which there's a film *(The Madness of King George)*, but a *crise de foie*? It seemed all the odder that such an alarmist—almost Pascalian—label should be given to a condition that clearly wasn't in the least life-threatening or physically incapacitating: hadn't the patient just walked in the door unaided?

So I did some reading. It's what Cecil Helman in his book *Culture, Health and Illness* calls a folk illness, a configuration of symptoms with no expression in biomedicine, and for which a culture provides both an explanation and a method of healing. There are other similarly tenacious folk illnesses across the world: *amok* in Malaysia, *windigo* in north-eastern America, *dil ghirda hai* ('sinking heart') in the Punjab, *brain fag* in parts of Africa, *nervios* in Latin America and *colds and chills* in the English speaking world.

Each condition exists in splendid isolation, marooned in its cultural uniqueness; and I wasn't a jot closer to understanding what a *crise de foie* was. Like every other medical complaint in France, it had its polypharmacy: strange elixirs containing 'oligoelements' in snap-open glass capsules and 'eupeptic' granulates to be taken *ante cibum* that were unknown to chemists in neighbouring countries. Before France started rationalising its drug formulary just a few years ago, at the end of the millennium, there were over one hundred preparations on the market for the fragile liver, most of which harked back to the nineteenth century. Fumbling his lines once in a chemist's shop in Paris, V. S. Pritchett in an amusing passage in his autobiography *Midnight Oil* tells us that instead of condoms he ended up with liver pills, and in a wild fit of 'faith and superstition' swallowed two before losing his virginity. As the great Canadian doctor Osler said, the real difference between humans and animals is that humans want to take pills.

Besides, that a symptom might be trivial is a value judgement not permitted a nation of amateur body theorists. As Colette Mechin says, 'you never tell a Frenchman he's suffering from indigestion, for that would give grounds for suspecting some dietary indiscretion'. Handle the French liver with caution: sensations of fullness, fleeting twinges and malaise may all be heralds of the great adversary.

But the symbolic weight carried by the French liver still wasn't obvious to me. Why should being liverish rather than being splenetic, say, be the *mal national*? Come to think of it, wasn't being liverish too literary, too poetic, to be much of a symptom? For me it was reminiscent of port decanters and portly gentlemen in one of Cruickshank or Rowlandson's merciless copperplate etchings of eighteenth-century English quacks and society characters.

Reading encyclopaedias can take you places where people speak far stranger languages than French even.

A patient with a *crise de foie* has the following symptoms: he feels bloated, has a thick head (but not necessarily headache), waterbrash (a bad taste in the mouth), lassitude and a general feeling of what Kafka once told his diary was 'seasickness on dry land'. It seems to resemble what most stolid folk would call a hangover (*gueule de bois* in vulgar French) and doctors dyspepsia, arriving like bad weather the morning after social surfeit. Surfeit entails disgust; and fatty foods are particularly contaminating and disgusting by virtue of their cloying properties.

Examination of such people is usually—as the phrase goes—unrevealing. My response is usually to show sympathy and tell him (nearly always a him) to take a couple of paracetamol and change his diet. *Primum non nocere.* Some doctors even stick—more out of curiosity than conviction, presumably—an acupuncture needle into the cure-all Liv 3 point which is on the dorsal side of the foot between the first two toes. The once famous moral tract *Traité de médecine générale* (still in print) recommends 'water only for 24 hours, vegetable broths, herbal teas, light meals, no alcohol and sleep', a regimen not likely to offend anybody's common sense. But I often have the impression that such a pragmatic response falls short of expectations, especially when the liver can excite such purple passages as this: 'Her *Shen* was low. This could be seen in the bronze colour of her face, the slightly rolled-back position of her eyeballs and her fatigued demeanour. Her pulse was wiry and rapid, indicating Uprising of Liver Fire syndrome' (*Acupuncture in Medicine* 11.96).

True enough, Chinese meridians make a big deal out of the liver. But what turns this little outpouching of entoderm, tucked above the yolk sac stalk, into the seat of humanity? In physiological terms, the liver is the body's (extremely efficient) sewage-plant, protein producer, and sugar and fat regulator. It's also the biggest organ, and its right-regal size may well explain its preponderance in cultural affairs. A 'critical liver' is a leftover from Galenic medicine, medieval theories of the spirits (in fact, Galen believed the liver was the receptacle of the 'natural' spirit, as opposed to the 'vital' and 'mental' spirits lurking in the heart and brain respectively), and Plato's suggestion in *Timaeus* that it was a divining mirror for cosmic space (chora); but while a recent evening-long search through Rabelais provided me with lots of extravagant remedies and nostrums, and the splendid line 'for I love you with all my liver', nothing very clearly emerged that might explain the quintessential liver in all its majesty, nor all the sublime hot air it has given rise to in French medicine. I therefore concluded that, French or otherwise, the liver is a signal instance of how we all think magically about our bodies. Not that our bodies are magical, but nobody, not even the most brick-headed enzymologist, is likely to view his liver in terms which exclude its miraculous ability to exempt him from toxic lapses. My own explanation therefore errs towards the Promethean.

Everyone remembers one thing about Prometheus ('fore-thinker'): he had such a rush of feeling for early man that he gave him a spark of fire he'd stolen from Zeus as it smouldered in a tube of fennel (a penis substitute, according to Freud, who thought that early man liked to snuff out fire by urinating on it). The myth is more intricate. Prometheus had been one of the assistants at the headbirth of Athena; later she'd taught him all the applied arts of civilisation including architecture, astronomy and navigation. Decently enough, he passed them on to the human creatures he so favoured.

It was an act of expediency that led to Prometheus' eventual downfall: he showed *Homo sapiens sapiens* how to trick Zeus by leaving him only the bones and gristle when the sacrificial animals were apportioned. After being called in to judge a dispute at Sicyon, in the north-eastern Peloponnese, Prometheus flayed an ox and made two bags of its skin; one containing all the prime cuts but with the tripe cunningly arranged on top (in the hierarchy of organs the stomach was always the lowest and most contemptible), the other the bones and gristle hidden under a layer of succulent fat. Zeus—'whose wisdom is everlasting'—chose as the divine share the bag with the layer of fat on top and bones beneath. He had been duped. All the edible meat had been left for the creatures Prometheus was bent on being kind to, except that Zeus arranged a subtle revenge: humans might get the 'better share' but it would always be accompanied by the demands of the stomach—that imperious, shameless, all-consuming organ. Humans would become meat-sacks, hollow bags that would have to be filled every day in order to sustain life. The imperiousness of hunger would empty all our more noble convictions and ideals and in times of neediness turn us into animals. We would become, in a word, appetites.

There is a coda to the myth, and a somewhat misogynistic one at that. Prometheus stole an ember from the sun-chariot and wrapped it in a fennel stalk for ready use at the ceremony of the barbecue. Humans might be condemned to eat meat, but at least they could cook it first. According to Hesiod, Zeus turned vindictive: he made the beautiful but simpering Pandora ('all gifts')—a gift being, as the German root-word alarmingly suggests, nothing other than poison—and sent her to Prometheus' seemingly slower-witted brother, Epimetheus ('afterthought'), whose name suggests that, like the chorus of a classical tragedy, his role was to bemoan the consequences of his brother's actions. Her receptacle contained all the spites and evils like Vice, Labour, Bipolar Disorders and Geriatric Infirmity that have subsequently plagued the world, and made necessary such lesser evils as doctors.

And once the spites had flown the jar and caused Pandora and Afterthinker nearly to die from anaphylactic shock, what was left? A booby-prize called Hope, which must have been heavier than air to get stuck inside; it was Hope that prevented their descendants, driven nearly out of their minds by the spites, from doing away with themselves. (The nineteenth-century German philosopher Arthur Schopenhauer once suggested that Hesiod got it completely wrong: it wasn't the evil but the *good* things of the world which flew away from Pandora's jar, leaving hope behind like a kind of miasmal slurry; and Friedrich Nietzsche tried to seal the jar again, precisely because for him hope *was* evil: it condemns what exists for something better.) *Prometheus pyrphoros*, the Fire-Carrier, ended up clamped to a rock in the Caucasus, his liver being pecked out daily by an eagle only for it to regenerate overnight—which sounds like the modern biomedical concept of the liver. Only the rock, insisted Franz Kafka in his minuscule fable about Prometheus' apprenticeship in suffering, is the really inexplicable part of the legend.

So much for Prometheus and the longwindedness of evolution, since the descendants of the eagle stopped pecking his liver and started nesting in his rib-cage, and Pandora's gift, it became clear in time, was a black box to tell us what had happened in the heroic days when the gods mixed it with humankind.

But the myth made me think of the French again, confused—as only a deeply conservative people can be—by their self-appointed role for the last few hundred years as the fire-carriers of modernity.

Progress is a no less exhausting idea than its opposite: to think our bodies a metaphor for the decrepitude of the world. A *crise de foie* must therefore be a kind of chronological vertigo—a morning's retributive visitation for sitting down the night before to sup nectar, in that sense of complete and utter well-being the French exude only at the dinner table, as if the *pays légal* ruled by Reason had given way to a *pays réel* of gastronomic abandon—Cockaigne or Schlaraffia—where the day's only order is the tripartite call to table. Botanising with their palates, as it were, in a world hermetically sealed against phasal eating stations, 'buns on the run' and the golden 'M'.

Yet gourmandising and apocalypse come together rather neatly in French consumptive habits, as seen to good effect in Marco Ferreri's painfully bulemic film *La grande bouffe* (1973), in which four men, in a parody of Jules Verne's voracious heroes, whose aim was that of 'eating everything, in impossible quantities, as often as possible', stuff themselves to death on every gastroglobal delicacy money can buy. Diagnosis? Fast food, slow food: myths are stratagems to enclose their opposites. And livers follow a cannibal logic. We have to sleep on them and they have to process those terrifying opposites, faith and doubt, which they do without fuss until dawn comes out, not rosy-fingered as Homer has it, but with a grey hair or two.

Now you know the answer to the biliously rhetorical question once posed as a title by the sociologist of terminal man, Jean Baudrillard. What are you doing after the orgy? Going to see the doctor, stupid.

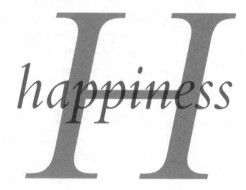

The Moral Life of Happiness

A GENEALOGY OF DIMINISHING RETURNS

The Western world has never been more prosperous than it now is, even if much of its wealth seems a futures trading version of the Biblical miracle of the loaves. What to former eras were utopian fantasies (greater productivity, reduced infant mortality, longer life expectancy) are now so taken for granted we hardly notice them. We only notice that reality is a more complicated and obscure matter than hitherto imagined when things refuse to bend to our imperious wills: this state of affairs is called a *scandal*. In the garden of earthly delights, market forces have even managed to turn hedonism into a kind of militancy. Yet journalists, sociologists and historians, Sigmund Freud and the occasional professional ethicist are equally of one voice: we are not happy. It is one of the distressing futilities at the heart of modern life, one related to that other contemporary concern: the less adversity we come up against the more we feel under threat.

But what is happiness, anyway? Why do we think it for the

asking when it more obviously steals upon us like a state of grace… or reveals itself only when our mood has ripened into regret? Why did some of the ancient Greek philosophers—and the idea *is* Greek—think happiness was a matter of having as few needs as possible? Are we too far gone in materialism to conceive of a neo-Platonic contemplator (Plotinus) asserting that even a person under torture can aspire to happiness? What inspired the German philosopher Nietzsche to write contemptuously of the Benthamite 'felicific calculus' (which, refined into the tenets of utilitarianism, has dominated so much thinking about social justice in the English-speaking world), 'man does not pursue happiness: only the Englishman does that'? Was it good sense or just a kind of cynical world-weariness that compelled François de la Roche-foucauld to write, 'We are never as happy nor as unhappy as we imagine.' And what led the poet W. H. Auden to insist in middle-age, in keeping with the providential arguments of an earlier age, that happiness is a *duty*? 'Be good and you will be happy is a dangerous inversion', he wrote. 'Be happy and you will be good is the truth.'

These are some of the questions that the London-based writer Ziyad Marar attempts to answer in his conceptual history of happiness, *The Happiness Paradox*, an invitation to meander through the author's stock of select quotations, urban legends, film plots, personal anecdotes and yarns. He starts with the shift in the term's freight in the middle of the eighteenth century. No longer did happiness signify a state of right living, less still the knowledge of being blessed in our lives—for the first time it made a gesture towards *feeling* good. Happiness had once served to describe the shape of an entire life (a largely miserable life could still be described as 'happy' if it was judged to be a *good* life); now it was fleet and punctual, a state more akin to gratification. By claiming in his *Discourse on Happiness* (1750) that happiness is a mental state dependent essentially on somatic conditions, La Mettrie—best known for his conflation of biology and mechanics—was able to redefine it primarily as a medical rather than an ethical issue. Happiness was losing its public dimension and becoming a sensation, internalised and self-spectating, even though it was still apparent to more reflective Enlightenment thinkers, such as Diderot, that the acceptance of a given social life had hitherto been the presupposition to there being moral judgements at all.

By the end of the eighteenth century, happiness could be actively sought, being congruent to the aspirations, and perhaps even to the acquisitive rhythm of life of the property-owning classes. La Mettrie's idea of man as a self-regulating machine was followed by Holbach's conception of happiness (felicity) as the condition to which humans, as physical beings, were entitled under the terms of the 'natural morality' he derived from the pleasure-principle and legislated for as the rule of social utility. ('Unnatural' morality was that imposed by the Christian religion, and further propagated by the political institutions of the *ancien régime*.)

After the French Revolution, the firebrand lawyer Saint-Just called happiness a new idea on earth, and tried to get it into people's heads by guillotining as many of them as possible—until he lost his own. It wasn't long before liberal writers like Stendhal were taking to the road in France and Italy in an attempt to find out just why happiness so rarely coincided with the desire that clamoured for it. Perhaps Stendhal ought to have stayed longer in England and more thoroughly wet his whistle, since, according to Dr Johnson, 'there is nothing which has yet been contrived by man, by which so much happiness is produced as by a good tavern'.

Part of the deeper problem was that the old concept of happiness as a social good had failed to disappear entirely: a market society might have no place for ordinary human sociability in its theoretical scheme of things, but mutuality is still necessary for the emotional economy of any society, perhaps most especially that of an egalitarian cargo-cult. Society is not simply a matter of relationships between persons; it is also the consciousness of those relationships in the minds of the individuals so related. Looking out for Number One can't help but become the focus of an unceasing manipulative tension.

So Marar's paradox is actually an *intensification*: it attaches to the fact that rather than having to legitimise himself before God the new individual has to justify himself before other men, which, as Jean-Jacques Rousseau complained most loudly and bitterly, is a kind of secular hell. Being modern means having to compare and be compared, to be saddled by the knowledge that there is no escape from having to plead, as did the Scottish poet Robert Burns, for the gift to see ourselves as others see us. We proclaim ourselves unique and irreplaceable, but that claim looks ridiculous when seen in the light of the equal claims of millions more. So we veer like weathervanes between the absurd solipsism of being 'self-made', and the abject plagiarism of prestigious others, a habit which advertises that the imitating acolyte hardly exists at all except by the force of his imitations. What could be more derivative or second-hand than cribbing from a model? What could be a better pretext for embarrassment, shame, humiliation and all the attendant self-conscious emotions?

'The modern sensibility both wants to break free and wants to belong', writes Marar. The more freedom we enjoy the less approval we receive; the more approval we seek the less free we become. His quasi-subjects are the latest biofeedback versions of La Mettrie's pleasure-pain machines, oscillating between the poles of control and remission. Acceptance of this polar condition offers, in his view, the perspective of understanding how going after happiness pulls us from 'disruption to conformity and back again'.

What he's not talking about is not an approximation to the old idea of the Golden Mean. Our societies are too creatively unstable, our economies too dependent on the cycle of appetites and disappointments, to allow that kind of harmony. Ultimate questions of what makes for the good life have been leached of sense in a civilisation predicated on the notion that a perpetual bounty of material goods is the best way to guarantee social peace: modern man has been trained to internalise a first-person doubt about all shared opinions, as well as to be seduced by the potentially illiberal thought that governments can and should guarantee his happiness.

The US Constitution guarantees, as Marar observes, the right to pursue happiness; it wisely refrains from saying anything at all about the nature of happiness itself. Carl Elliot, an American bioethicist, takes the view, in his tolerant and mildly ironic book *Better than Well*—the latest instalment in a modern tradition examining America's obsession with therapy that began with Tom Wolfe's 1973 essay 'The Me Decade'—that the contemporary eagerness for the technological fixes offered by medicine has less to do with consumerism's infantile prospects of instant gratification than a touch of personal evangelism: the desire to be fulfilled. To be fulfilled in America is to be a self-respecting and respectable social actor. It is to be a puritan once the original premises of Puritanism have been forgotten.

If happiness is a duty that takes the form, especially after the 1960s, of 'an obligation to the self', then the self-attending individual is bound to get anxious about being seen to be so beholden to others. Authenticity is at stake, and the very spontaneity of desire. In a society of individualists nobody dare admit to being a conformist. Indeed, the only nobility in a world where looking foolish (being made to look foolish) is the basic fact of social existence is awareness of the fact itself, and its strategic use to deflate the condition that imposes it: Dostoevsky writes about almost nothing else.

Elliott's chapters offer a thought-provoking tour around his theoretical speculations, moving from a consideration of the pioneering American sociologist Thorstein Veblen (who came up with the term 'conspicuous consumption' as long ago as 1899) to such phenomena as the post-war rise of depression as a clinical diagnosis, short-lived psychiatric syndromes like fugue state and repressed memory, the new phenomenon of 'apotemnophilia' (apotemnophiliacs are otherwise well people who go to any lengths, including self-mutilation, to become amputees: these are individuals whose *felt* integrity can be had only through loss of their actual *physical* integrity), and the various kinds of surgical and drug-based treatments that promise to transform what would formerly have been thought unchangeable aspects of human personality and identity. 'Why is loneliness not / A chemical discomfort…?' queried Auden in a poem of 1960, anticipating by thirty years the assumption behind the latest generation of serotonin reuptake inhibitor drugs. Elliott suggests that if Americans worry about these treatments, as suggested by the loaded term 'enhancement technologies' (which draws attention to their *transformative* potential while obscuring the fact that some may be quite conventional treatments of the *restorative* kind), it is largely because they worry about 'the good life these technologies serve'. Once the purview of medicine gets extended to boosting a person's sense of well-being, then the scope of potentially treatable conditions can only expand enormously.

Elliott cites Wittgenstein's famous thought experiment of the community of language-users with a 'beetle in a box', in which every person claims to know what a beetle is by examining only his own box, and has no right to peek into his neighbour's—a logical parable to show that what has a public dimension cannot be private, and that what *is* private cannot be a language—as a mechanism for the seeding of doubt about status in a democratic society; and the need to keep up with the Joneses. Are other people playing by the rules of the game or pulling a fast one? Desire is not a democracy; it establishes new hierarchies. Elliott is describing not so much people playing a game but the world of Stendhal's tormented and deadly serious *vaniteux*. Our world of escalating wants is the result.

While the American sense of endlessly manipulable well-being is spreading with the global market, a sense of diminishing possibility fed to Europeans by their historical sixth sense (not so much vestigial as undeveloped, we are led to believe, among Americans) has long made us experts in self-mutilation: our apotemnophilia is all at the symbolic level, which is of course where it really hurts. Good Europeans have never aspired to be happy: Freud's goal was to minimize suffering, and psychoanalysis, at least to begin with, offered a kind of negative freedom. It taught members of the middle classes how to cope with the solitude produced by a market society.

Germany is a case in point. The great nineteenth-century Prussian novelist Theodor Fontane wrote, 'the large city has no time for thinking and, what is worse, it has no time for happiness. What it creates a hundred times over is the Hunt for Happiness, which is actually the same as unhappiness.' Such perspicuity notwithstanding, it is a terrible historical irony that the nightmare history that followed the attempts of the Nazis to fabricate a happy utopia based on exclusion has meant that more recently in Fontane's country happiness was once called—no doubt with polemic intent—a *crime*. This position, the vigilant reader will realise, is the switch-side of the Marquis de Sade's.

The greatest achievement of Elliott's book, which draws purposefully on literature, history, sociology and anthropology, is to show just how some trends in society demand to be examined not in the standard quantitative Benthamite mode but as an extended essay in the manner of Montaigne (who has a chapter in his *Essays* that bears the Aristotelian title, 'That we should not be deemed happy till after our death.'). Elliott's book bears comparison with some of the best essay writing on contemporary American society—even if it neglects to say much about the deeper historical influences on American ideas of happiness.

Rousseau, for instance, is the torchbearer for America's recurrent sense of itself as an *innocent* county; and his dream of being a new Adam prior to the troubling claims of adult civilisation could very profitably have been brought into the discussion. 'One must be true to oneself; that is the homage which the honest man must pay to his own dignity.' Call self-fulfilment *righteousness*, and the essentially religious nature of happiness crops up again, except that morality is a blunt thing in a society that ostentatiously rejects what some of its citizens complain it lacks: a sense of limit and constraint.

Such is the peculiarity of consumerist America: it has liberalism as its orthodoxy and not its radicalism, as in Europe, while retaining all the self-righteous fervour of a dissenting religious utopia. Neither Elliott nor Marar, being thoroughly schooled in the cultural sociology of luminaries like Erving Goffman, devote much attention to the mechanisms of the market, which are credited as never before with being able to maintain social peace by their ability to deliver the goods—even though these same mechanisms are manifestly in the dark about human wants (unless we want to credit the Invisible Hand of the market with godlike rectitude). As Robert Reich argues in *The Future of Success*, market society is always threatened by the success of its own productivity, which, if it were to satisfy our needs in the innocently self-evident way that befell the great minds of the eighteenth-century ('Enlightenment in all classes of society really consists in correctly grasping the nature of our essential needs': Georg Christoph Lichtenberg, 1789) would be bound to put itself out of business. It therefore has to skew our regard towards things we can never have enough of. Thus are values swallowed up by desire, which in the end seeks nothing very concrete at all.

But that would be to lurch into metaphysics, and the company of the types Nietzsche suggested were even more contemptible than the Englishman. He calls them 'the last men'. They have made any kind of criticism a sin, and happiness the outcome of a state-sponsored population strategy. They indulge their little pleasures for day and night, 'but they respect health'. For these last men the old world was quite obviously barking mad. 'We have discovered happiness', they tell his prophet Zarathustra. And then they blink, in the terrifyingly guileless spirit of that line in Alexander Pope's poem *Eloisa to Abelard*—in the eternal sunshine of the spotless mind.

Observing the distracted state of my contemporaries sometimes convinces me that Nietzsche foresaw the nature of the last men all too accurately. But in fact the dictionary provides a remedy for despair. The etymology of the word 'happiness' belies the prospect of its ever being *planned*: its Middle English cognates—chance, hap, luck—are terms for what is not designed or projected. Happiness has no recipe. It cannot be engineered, as in the mixed-register phrase Jane Austen artfully uses in *Emma* to describe one of her pushy characters, dressed in 'all her apparatus of happiness'. It is the contrary of the deal offered by the prudent evangelisers who seek to protect us from risks. In fact, it has most to do with another word that also answers to those three cognates: *adventure*. Happiness is a dare.

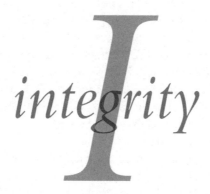

integrity

An Empty Plot

In the small hours of Monday 11 January, 1993, Luc Ladmiral, a general practitioner in Voltaire-Ferney, a dormitory town for Geneva on the French side of the border, received a call to say that the house of his best friend in the neighbouring town was in flames. When he got there the firemen were in the process of bringing out the charred remains of the two children, Antoine (five) and Caroline (seven), and their mother Florence. Only Jean-Claude Romand, the father, still showed signs of life. He was rushed away in an ambulance, unconscious, to a burns unit across the Swiss border.

Both men had been friends for nearly twenty years, since university; both were doctors; they had married almost at the same time; their children had grown up together; Luc's eldest child was Jean-Claude's goddaughter. And now this. A boiler had caught fire in the night, and a family had been destroyed. In the still of the early morning, the distraught Ladmirals prayed together that

Jean-Claude would never come round from his coma.

When Luc opened his surgery later that morning two policemen were waiting to speak to him. The three victims of the fire had actually been murdered, the children shot, the mother's skull staved in. On going to break the awful news to Jean-Claude's parents in the hamlet of Clairvaux-les-Lacs, in the Jura, his uncle had found the house silent. They too had been shot, along with their dog. The police asked Luc what he knew about Jean-Claude's life outside his family. Did he have any enemies? Debts? Suspicious activities? They wanted to know more about his post as a researcher at the World Health Organization.

Luc knew very little about his friend's professional life. Jean-Claude had always been the soul of discretion and modesty, adept at showing others in their best light. His wife proudly told her friends he was a 'superdoctor', working quietly away in a neon-lit lab in Geneva to make all those wonderful treatments possible (although this is not what the bureaucrats at WHO do at all). Yet there was no official record of Romand on the WHO staff list. Nor was his name registered with the regional medical council. The Paris hospitals where he claimed to have done his internship had ever heard of him. Most oddly of all, there was no trace at all of him as a graduate of the University of Lyon Nord, where he and Luc had trained. There had to be some mistake: this was his best friend. Hadn't they gone through medical school together?

A note, a confession of sorts, was found in Romand's car; it referred to an 'injustice' connected with his children's school. Someone had wanted to 'punch his face in' after a dispute at a board meeting. Surely this couldn't be a reason to massacre a family? Then a former lover, a divorcee who had once lived near Ferney, phoned the police. Romand had met her in Paris on the Saturday evening (the autopsies showed that the family had been killed that morning) in order to escort her—so she believed—to dinner at Fontainebleau with Bernard Kouchner, founder of Médecins sans Frontières and one of Romand's supposed big-name friends; on the way he had attacked and tried to strangle her. She had asked him to return the savings of 900 000 francs which she had invested through him, at an advantageous rate of interest, in a Swiss account. In fact, he had embezzled the money, hers being the last in a series of nest-eggs sucked dry in order to fund his middle-class lifestyle. Nobody, it seems, had ever asked him for receipts. A million francs had come from his wife's family to supplement what he had already dispensed of his parents' capital; now questions were being asked about the death of Romand's father-in-law several years before, after a fall down a staircase while alone in the house with his son-in-law.

Three days after being rescued from his burning house, Romand came to. He was suffering from the effects of smoke inhalation and the barbiturates he had taken before setting the house on fire after his return from Paris. The police began a detailed investigation, and the newspapers had a field day. Having first read about the murder that week, on the day he finished his biography of the science fiction writer Philip K. Dick (a somewhat dysfunctional personality himself), Emmanuel Carrère, cult writer, *père de famille* and connoisseur of parallel worlds, finally decided that the only person who could answer the questions that had begun to trouble him was Romand himself. Six months after the murder he wrote to Romand in jail: 'I should like you to understand that I am not approaching you out of some unhealthy curiosity or a taste for the sensational. What you have done is not in my eyes the deed of a common criminal nor that of a madman but the action of someone pushed to the limit by overwhelming forces, and it is these terrible forces I would like to show at work.' Along with his flattering concession that Romand might be the victim rather than the villain of the piece, Carrère sent a copy of his new Dick biography, realising only after posting it that the title might not be an altogether happy one in the circumstances: *I Am Alive and You Are Dead*.

Two years later, having meanwhile written a baleful novel about a murderous father (published in English as *Class Trip*) and having almost forgotten his obsession, Carrère received a reply from the prison in Bourg-en-Bresse. Romand had read his novel; he recognised himself in the child it portrayed; he was keen to co-operate. Thrown into a quandary, Carrère decided he would reply. There followed an odd exchange of letters, Carrère adopting a deferential tone because of his 'guilt about not being guilty', Romand dilating on the meaning of his suffering (he had begun reading Lacan). He sent Carrère a clipping from a psychiatrist's report: 'he was part of them and they of him in a cosmogonic system that was all-embracing, undifferentiated and closed. At that level, there is no longer much difference between suicide and murder.' Carrère's intervention in his life was 'a sign': he was counting on the writer to explain his story to him better than the psychiatrists had been able to.

The trial was set for June 1996. Carrère went off for a week to visit the places where Romand had played out his double life, with an itinerary which had been drawn up by the murderer himself. He saw the hamlet in the Jura where Romand had grown up as the withdrawn single son of a forester, the burned-down house in Prévessin, the parents' cottage in the woods. It was a desolate experience. 'And here I was again, chosen (a strong term, I know, but I don't see how I can say it any other way) by that atrocious story, drawn within the orbit of a man who had done *that*. I was afraid. Afraid and ashamed. Ashamed in front of my children, that their father should be writing about that.' All of France's crime reporters were at the trial. 'It's not every day you get to see the face of the Devil', commented *Le Monde*. Catching sight of the strained faces of Florence's family, Carrère realises he is *parti pris* for the accused: 'It was to him that I felt I owed consideration because, wishing to tell this story, I saw it as *his* story.'

The story which unfolded in the courtroom was a conventional enough one for a bright country boy growing up in a quiet part of the rural France that had been transformed by the country's post-war boom: France's flight from the land occurred in living memory. The Romands had been foresters in the Jura for generations, were almost a clan; his father, Aimé, was a timber manager, respected in the trade: a man of probity, quiet and undemonstrative. His mother Anne-Marie worried constantly, and often took to her bed, so Jean-Claude learned to 'mislead' her so as not to make her worry even more. Emotions were considered a caprice in the family, whose motto ran: a Romand tells the truth and shames the Devil. That left white lies: 'And when you get caught in that endless effort not to disappoint people,' he explained to the presiding judge, 'the first lie leads to another, and then it's your whole life.'

He was an exemplary *lycien*. He received top marks in the first part of his baccalaureate exam. His parents wanted him to follow in the family line of business; he admired his father and had a real love of the forest. So in order to cram for the Forestry Commission's competitive examination, he went to a preparatory class in Lyon, arriving—if Carrère is to be believed—like some kind of Kaspar Hauser among the snobbish sons of the middle-class for whom a forester was a *plouc*—a hick. It was a breach with his background and Jean-Claude suddenly felt a need to climb the social ladder. He announced to his family that he wanted to study medicine, although what might have seemed to be a young man striking out on his own was actually the reverse. He had never had the slightest interest in patients, he later told Carrère, and the thought of touching bodies was repellent to him. He was paying obeisance to a social idol. Yet rather than being taken aback or disappointed by his decision, his parents were delighted: Aimé's son, the village boy, was making good.

At the Lyon-Nord medical faculty, he got to know Florence, a distant cousin. She was a down-to-earth, straightforward girl who seemed destined for an uneventful life. Soon it was understood that they were a couple, though Florence was notably reluctant to embark on the relationship; he was a big lad, and a bit flabby and unprepossessing. Together they were part of a clique that included Luc Ladmiral. Then the big lie happened, the crucial failure of will, the event that led, insanely but logically, to all the others. He failed to turn up for his crucial second-year exam, the 'barrage' for clinical placements, and though he could have saved face in a number of ways he told his parents he'd been accepted into the third year. He'd run smack into a dead-end, as Carrère says, even before he'd started out. 'How could he have suspected that there was something worse than being quickly unmasked, which was *not* to be unmasked, so that this childish lie would lead him eighteen years later to murder his parents, Florence, and the children he did not yet have?'

He spent that first term shut up in a studio apartment his parents had bought him. Weeks went by before Luc managed to get through to him, having assumed that his absence was due to a quarrel with Florence. What was wrong? Instead of coming clean, Jean-Claude let the lie metastasise. He told Luc he had a Hodgkin's lymphoma, a tumour of uncertain prognosis which allowed life to continue more or less normally, but was liable to flare up unpredictably. Luc had to promise not to tell Florence. Jean-Claude patched up his relationship with Florence, and got a doctor to sign a certificate to explain his absence from the exam. Soon he was expertly manipulating the anonymity of French university bureaucracy: for twelve years, he registered as a second-year student, thereby obtaining a student ID card and a letter stating that he was not eligible to sit the entrance exam in September, a charade which continued until 1986 when a new dean asked the phantom student to visit her in person. (Student status was a useful let-out from having to pay income tax, one later supplanted by his new identity as an international civil servant.) He tagged along to classes with his friends, used the library, photocopied the same notes: in short, did everything they were doing in order to become the genuine article. Florence had failed the second-year exam, and decided to study pharmacology, so they weren't in the same classes anymore, but that didn't stop them studying together. Jean-Claude was bright and ambitious; Florence thought he would go far. He avoided the small clinical teaching groups and of course the exams, though he was often to be seen mingling in the nervously chattering crowd outside the hall. Nobody noticed he didn't actually go in.

Romand put more energy into being a sham doctor than he would have done into being a real one. That might be the prerogative of the true con artist; but Romand seemed to have derived no secret pleasure from his act of deception. He went off to Paris, ostensibly to prepare for the competitive training exams, and then told everyone he had bagged a post as a researcher in Lyon. Soon he and Florence had settled in Voltaire-Ferney, which was an ideal location for his next job: at the Geneva headquarters of the World Health Organization. The children were born, Caroline ('Caro') and Antoine ('Titou'). Romand never invited colleagues home, never put on airs. He didn't want the children to think they were anything special. Indeed, he refused to be disturbed at work: not even his wife had his office number. An answering service relayed calls to him. It seems a shaky facade, but nobody ever shook it to see if it held. Every morning he dropped his children off at school, and then drove to the WHO carpark. Sometimes he used the ground-floor facilities such as the bank or travel bureau, but never ventured to the higher levels where security was tighter. That was in the beginning; then he moved on to sitting in cafés, reading the papers, or walking aimlessly through the forest to kill time. On Thursdays he supposedly lectured in Dijon. He would fake overseas trips, holing out in the airport hotel before returning home to complain about jet-lag. He made a point of bringing appropriate presents for the children.

What finally brought about the implosion was his defence of the headmaster at the school, who had been dismissed after having an affair with another teacher. He drew attention to himself in the community; for the first time 'he had said what he thought'. For the first time he was also under real pressure: his former mistress in Paris wanted her money back. One week before the murder of his family the president of the school board met Florence in the street and told her he couldn't find her husband's name in the internal WHO directory. Then Jean-Claude's mother telephoned, upset that the bank had sent a letter reporting a substantially overdrawn account. He promised to see to it, reassuring her that it must have been a mistake. Later that week he obtained a bottle of phenobarbitol solution from the local pharmacy, no questions asked. In a weapons store, he purchased a silencer and cartridges. Later in the week he filled some canisters with petrol.

Carrère is like one of those 'no apparatus' divers who practise the extreme brinkmanship of getting themselves winched down into very deep water, while retaining just enough air in the lungs to prevent fatal loss of consciousness on the way up. Despite this spell of self-induced apnoeia, he manages a very sober style. It is one that wraps itself in an atmosphere of grey nightmare, though his willingness to suspend judgement and let the narrative drag him down suggests a dangerous degree of identification with this terribly modern story of posture and imposture. There is no floor to Romand's personality (although one of the examining psychiatrists does say it—'Jean-Claude would have made an excellent psychiatrist'), no plane on which motive might relate to deed. All writers suffer from the apparent wastage of days, and may even attempt to make free with necessity: if Carrère writes with more than the usual guilt, it must be in the knowledge that his book will be conscripted as one of the narratives Romand uses to reconstruct the meaning of a life of which he, the man with the ominous name, woefully refused to be author.

The most unsettling moment in Carrère's account occurs when he decides to visit the Jura and explore the setting of the subterfuge for himself: he gets sucked into a time-warp. The sense of dread he conveys is more authentic than any emotion experienced by his subject—it is a loss of self, of connection to the world. Liars try too hard to be plausible, which is what gives them away; Romand—'the big baby'—was radically thoughtless. He had stopped thinking in that fateful second year of medical school.

Carrère shuns forensic speculation: had he written a standard clinical biopic of a sociopath with obscurely Oedipal fears and a narcissistic sense of his own worth, we would have had a far less compelling story. He notes that, in prison, Romand has acquired a newly abject identity as 'the lowest possible thing in society' and with the support of some enthusiastic Catholic prison visitors '"condemned himself to live" so as to dedicate his suffering to his family's memory'. This, he suspects, can only be another form of self-deception, the work of the 'adversary' of the novel's title, Satan, who is first mentioned explicitly at that terrible moment when Romand betrays his parents' trust. Satan could be more pointedly understood as the force behind the social order as idol. If Romand was possessed by anything it was the passively biddable demon of conformism. Dostoevsky would have recognised the type instantly. The literary critic and anthropologist René Girard spells out its effects: 'Satan could be said to incarnate mimetic desire were that desire not, by definition, disincarnated. It empties all people, all things, and all texts of their substance.' The young boy from the woods who hasn't woken up to the nature of responsibility chooses the one profession that might put him beyond reproach: medicine. Altruism is twinned with egoism, or recruited as a kind of immunity against its effects. Moving into adulthood seems to have been a peculiar degradation for Romand. If being a man means being an actor (Gombrowicz), then all it took for him to be a doctor was to impersonate one. He counterfeited the virtues. And it was his overriding need to protect this idealised self from being unmasked in front of those to whom it might conceivably have mattered that finally led him to murder. In Robert Louis

Stevenson's famous novella, Dr Jekyll surrenders the integrity of his person for the sake of that other 'integrity', a spotless reputation. He ends up not so much ensnared by his shadow-double, Hyde, as having ceased to be anybody at all.

While another contemporary novel comes to mind on reading *The Adversary*, not just because of the affectless tone they have in common, Georges Perec's 'infra-ordinary' first novel *Things* (1965), a critical take on France's emerging consumer society in which two characters are tracked on their travels around France and Tunisia, its geographical setting suggests a much older precursor. It unfolds in that part of the world where Jean-Jacques Rousseau, having abandoned any hope of recovering natural man, tormented himself with the distinction between *amour de soi*, a healthy self-preserving instinct, and its corrupting double, *amour-propre* or self-esteem, an invidious feeling derived from comparison with others, an emotion both relative and reactive. He was defining the terms for the theatre of duplicity we all inhabit. Concerning everything which touched him in the mobile prison of his paranoia—whether politics, education, or relationships—Rousseau kept lancing himself with the one question: why do things go wrong? Moral progress can only be assessed by criteria whose authority is external to personal desire: if choice alone is authoritative, then the individual is playing a game that is arbitrary and self-enclosed (hence the importance for Rousseau of the general will).

It is certainly remarkable that another explorer of selfhood, Friedrich Nietzsche—whose term for *amour-propre* was 'the will to power'—should pen a maxim that describes the protagonist of Carrère's book with uncanny accuracy: 'The most dangerous doctors are those born actors who imitate born doctors with perfect deceptive art.'

The Gex region, where Romand set up home, straddles one of Europe's internal borders. Borders can be stimulating places for those of no fixed allegiance, but they also provide cover for people like Romand. His fiscal identity was smoothly adapted to his fiction, so long as it lasted. Strasbourg, where I live, offers a parallel: not only does it boast the highest density of psychiatrists in any French city, some of them bent on solving the eternal question about how Alsace, which is culturally Alemannic (middle high

German), belongs to the 'one and indivisible' French republic; it also has quires of bureaucrats prone to the kind of 'holier than thou' moral exhibitionism that only the administration of human rights, it seems, can generate these days. The existence in Geneva of a transnational organisation impersonally working for the common good made it possible for Romand to style himself a minor Schweitzer even though the job he said he was doing had nothing at all to do with real patients. Abstract piety allowed him to play the contemporary double-bluff: individualism and bureaucracy need each other however much they hate to admit it. And we are all implicated insofar as we choose to pursue a specialised form of knowledge and then allow that specialisation to blind us to the order of reality we actually inhabit. Literature knows this dilemma better than society; Carrère's book hints at a problem that has leaked out of aesthetics and infected the social world. Although he refused to recognise that a lie—*his* lie—could ever be a sufficient cause, Romand grasped with near perfect deceptive art how to protect what looked like autonomy; and when the façade cracked, he was prepared, as R. D. Laing put it in *The Divided Self*, to abandon everything dear to him except the fortress of his inner self, even though it had been an echo chamber for years.

This demoralising story of harm and deprivation is a relic of the mood that descended on France in the 1990s, when the pressures of the global market threatened to turn the country's never very solid civic institutions into a franchise in which self-determination was the sole measure of social legitimacy and the rule of law the only buffer to egoism. It is as if, for Carrère at least, the slogan of May 1968, *sous les pavés—la plage*, has flattened out into the vision of Romand's null existence as he drives round the countryside: 'a vast beach of dead and empty time'.

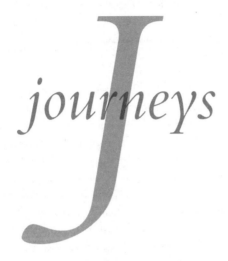

journeys

Chekhov Goes to Sakhalin

A WORKING HOLIDAY IN A PENAL INSTITUTION

Of all the great nineteenth-century literary figures, Chekhov is one of the few not to have had his reputation debunked. This may be because he did the job himself: a travel-book about Siberia?—a far-fetched literary gag indeed.

In early 1890 Alexei Suvorin, newspaper tycoon, editor of *Novoye Vremya* (*New Times*) and sponsor for the trip to Sakhalin, the prison colony off the pacific coast of Russia north of Japan which, with its mean annual temperature of zero Celsius, rude geography and ten months of winter, was a cold, inhospitable place to sustain any kind of reforming programme, wrote to Chekhov in bafflement—'no one needs Sakhalin, and it possesses no interest for anybody'. Chekhov replied, in a tone of feigned affront, that his work would yield nothing for literature or science, although he wished to repay medicine 'towards which [...] I have been a real swine', and that in any case he 'had been growing indolent for some time now' and really had to take himself in hand.

Convinced? Chekhov wasn't. He concedes, 'none of this is convincing', and then asserts, jauntily: 'personally I'm going out there for the most trivial of reasons'. It was as if, to quote from *A Boring Story,* written not long before he hatched the Sakhalin scheme, he was about to acquire the 'ability to preserve his dignity on a wild-goose chase'.

Sakhalin is off the map, a fleck on the flank of Asia. The island had officially become Russian territory after a dispute with the Japanese in 1875, though the Russian government had long been sending convicts there. Tundra over much of its northern half, forested with spruce, birch and pine in the south, this long mountainous backbone in the sea of Okhotsk is about as far away from Moscow within Russia as Chekhov could get: 5000 miles. And it wasn't just that. Chekhov's decision to go overland—the first sleepers for the Trans-Siberian Railway would be sunk ten years later—rather than follow the usual shipping route from Odessa around the coast of Asia (which is how everyone got there, except the chain-gangs) is just as odd as deciding to go at all. He seems to be making an ordeal out of an epic: the Great Siberian Highway was little better than an unsealed dirt track.

Opting for sackcloth and ashes, even if only for the space of a summer vacation, would have been too much like his childhood in Taganrog to appeal to Chekhov; and it is difficult to match the self-imposed rigours of a coach journey to Siberia with the philosophy of idleness he espoused but never practised until his tuberculosis made it unavoidable: 'My ideal: to be idle, and love a fat girl.'

Chekhov had no legal qualifications, and he was certainly not a bleeding-heart liberal. If anything, he tended to mock 'do-gooders'; he steered clear of the vocal, politically radical faction in the Moscow literary scene and disliked the often crudely stereotypic way Enlightenment and Reaction were portrayed in contemporary novels. Although he'd been writing since his student days, Chekhov's own claim to be a serious writer was at best a few years old: his collection *In the Twilight* was published in 1887 and his most ambitious story *The Steppe* had appeared in a 'thick journal', the Petersburg monthly *Severny vestnik* (*The Northern Herald*) in

March 1888. Much of the 'eighties had in fact been taken up with what he called 'balderdash'—captions and advertisements, gossipy sketches of street life, comic calendars, literary parodies, questionnaires and even a detective novel. Chekhov was writing for the newly literate clerks and those who, like himself, took the train from Melikhovo, where he purchased a small estate in 1892, to the capital.

Of all his published fiction, 528 items—not including his weekly gossip column and other occasional journalism—were written between 1880 and the watershed year 1888; a mere 60 would be written in the remaining sixteen years of his life.

Contemporary events don't clarify motives either. Chekhov had been deeply shaken by the 'white plague' from which his brother Nikolai ('Kolia') died in June 1889 and sister-in-law Anna the year before; and six of his medical year were to succumb to cholera and typhus epidemics around the same time. Torpor and morosity might have been more easily understandable. His own health, too, was increasingly undermined by paroxysms of coughing and bouts of haemoptysis, telltale signs of the TB that was formally diagnosed only in 1897 (and from the complications of which he died in 1904). Regarding which, his insouciance seems flip and forced: his letter to Suvorin of 1888 is a classic in denial of a peculiarly professional kind—'by itself, haemorrhaging from the lungs is not significant...'

In the background was Tolstoy, his literary Moses. Tolstoy had cast something of a spell over Chekhov from the mid-1880s; he had been involved, as a precedent, in the visit to the wretched residents of the Lyapin and Rzhanov Lodging Houses that he describes in *What Then Must We Do?* (1886). No book, perhaps, has better exposed the unhappy relationship between philanthropy and pity in action. Resenting the contempt of the housekeeper who supposedly looks after them, Tolstoy's words in defence of the prostitutes suddenly brings the place to life, in a scene he compares with Ezekiel's field of bones quivering at the touch of the spirit (a Biblical image that crops up too in the final paragraph of the final volume of Charles Booth's massive statistical survey of poverty in Victorian London); and yet their expectation of his saying more—'as though they had only been waiting for that word to cease to be corpses and to become alive'—suddenly makes him feel fraudulent. Abashed, he can say nothing at all.

'Only a very unhappy man', wrote Wittgenstein, 'has the right to pity someone else.'

Tolstoy's grip on the younger writer was on the wane before Sakhalin, but the journey may be seen as the final shadow cast by that influence. Yet Chekhov cheerfully neglects Tolstoyan principles throughout the journey; in his letters to his family he worries about running out of cigarettes or vodka, and from the shores of Lake Baikal complains to his sister Masha about the lack of fresh meat and liquor. A philosophy of self-reliance must have seemed an armchair absurdity to Chekhov in Siberia, where settlers either depended on each other or didn't depend at all. The son of a shopkeeper who went bankrupt when he was sixteen, Chekhov had few illusions about the appeal to Tolstoy of what were, in effect, noble savages. 'Muzhik [peasant] blood flows in my veins,' Chekhov commented apropos of Tolstoy's idealising of the Russian peasantry, 'and you can't astonish me with muzhik virtues.' The peasants he writes about after his return are drunk, flatly unimprovable, aggressively themselves, and have none of the extenuating character traits or dubious *sancta simplicitas* attributed to them by the older writer.

'Devil take the great philosophies of this world!' was how he dismissed the subject of the Russian soul; and he admitted to Suvorin that Tolstoy's *The Kreutzer Sonata*—which he had thought a great book before he left for Sakhalin—now seemed 'ridiculous and incoherent'. It exposed Tolstoy, in his opinion, 'as an ignorant man who has never at any point in his long life taken the trouble to read two or three books written by specialists'. The difference between them is apparent in their attitude to medicine: although he never romanticised science in the grand style like Pasteur or Pavlov, Chekhov had hopes for the future of his profession and remained a meliorist about social progress.

The sage of Yasnaya Polyana, on the other hand, thought doctors were scoundrels who put cleanliness before godliness. Chekhov would be a better writer, he once remarked to Gorki, if medicine didn't stand in his way.

The rebuttal of Tolstoy's moralistic agenda for the ascetic life is developed in his short story *Ward No. 6*, written a couple of years after Sakhalin, when Chekhov was busy helping to build new schools on his estate at Melikhovo and doing a fair bit of doctoring on the side—much like Dr Pascal in Zola's novel, which was serialised in Russia in 1893. *Ward No. 6* offers a critique of the doctrine of non-resistance to evil: Dr Andrei Yefimich Ragin is committed to his own mental ward after he becomes the victim of an ambitious colleague's intrigue.

The story's turning point is Ragin's acknowledgement of something he had been staring at for years without ever noticing it: his patients have feelings—dear God, even *he* has feelings! Monotony and futility have evidently taken their toll on Dr Ragin, who initially began his career in this provincial hospital as a diligent and purposeful practitioner. He has allowed the hospital to go to seed; retreated from his duties; guarded patients rather than treated them.

One day, a thirty-three-year-old man named Gromov, incarcerated because of his persecution mania, stirs Ragin's interest. For the first time, he has extended conversations with a patient. Gromov bluntly points out to him that doctors don't know much about suffering since they attempt to understand objectively something that can only be felt. They live, if they live at all, vicariously. 'Why, it's so obvious! The man's a doctor and doesn't even know a little thing like that! Contempt for suffering, permanent contentment, never being surprised… it just means sinking to *that* condition.' Ragin is a Pharisee exposed, the hypocrite who tells patients how virtuous it is to be stoical.

He takes to visiting the 'mad ward' daily, not because Gromov's words have cut him to the quick but because he finds their chats 'original'. After twenty years of not visiting his patients, this departure from the routine is enough to get tongues wagging elsewhere in the hospital. Asked to 'take a holiday', he is finally tricked into entering the asylum by his successor. Dr Ragin is now a patient himself.

Chekhov makes this change in status utterly believable, and absolutely comfortless. For it is only after being punched in the face by the orderly whose casual brutality he had for so long tolerated (and who used to call him 'Your Excellency') that Ragin grasps the grim reality of his situation; the next day he is dead of a stroke. Russia's supine history is in that story, wrote a certain Vladimir Ulianov, who as a young revolutionary thought he himself had been locked up in Ward 6.

Thomas Mann wrote that Chekhov's argument with Tolstoy had forced the former to raise irony to open rebellion.

Chekhov's instinct was not misplaced: he had to extend himself physically, in an absurdly pedestrian manner, in order to win clarity for himself as a writer. A frail Gogol travels on a hazardous expedition to Jerusalem, in 1848, in search of inspiration; a hardly more robust Chekhov skirts the pot-holes on the road to Sakhalin. His trip in fact cost him the best part of his health. No other piece of writing posed him such difficulties: he spent nearly four years revising his account, and his earnings took a dive, since his absence from the Moscow scene deprived him of literary and medical income.

Yet if anything was ever going to count in backward Russia, it was the work of individuals. There are still things to do in the world, he tells his friends. Who were his models? Not the great thinkers. Chekhov was fascinated by men of action; with the African explorers and Stanley's *In Darkest Africa* in particular. The 1880s was the decade of unbridled European enthusiasm for adventure in Africa, the decade Germany got the 'African bug' and infected by *Torschlusspanik*—fear of missing the bus—started out on its own imperial enterprise, while giving the go-ahead to the cruellest imperial farce of all: Leopold II's 'humanitarian' project in the Congo Basin, the backdrop to Conrad's *Heart of Darkness*.

In 1888, Chekhov had written an enthusiastic unsigned obituary of Nikolai Przhevalsky, the explorer of China and Tibet and the discoverer of Przewalski's horse, for *New Times*: his imagination was fired by the spectacle of the explorer who had abandoned his family and died in harness, by a remote lake on the Kirgizian border. 'When European societies are seized by indolence,' he had written, 'heroes are as necessary as the sun.'

All of which suggests a rather different Chekhov from the well-mannered, distant writer who chimes the dinner gong in the Gardens of the West—this is a Boy's-own Chekhov. His journey to Sakhalin, which gets only a passing mention in many older biographies, controverts the standard view of him, in D. S. Mirsky's words, as someone who completely rejected 'what we may call the heroic values'. It makes him, rather piquantly, god-father to the humanitarian grand gesture which has absorbed so many of Europe's disaffected, idealistic or unemployed doctors since 1968, the kind of publicity-hungry NGO action associated with a group like Médecins sans Frontières.

Having set his mind on going to Sakhalin, and more or less convinced his family and friends that he really had no choice in the matter, Chekhov prepared himself thoroughly. He read over a hundred publications on the island and the penal system, as well as books on botany, geography and tiresome government reports. He writes to Pleshcheyev: 'All day I sit reading and making extracts. In my head and on paper there is nothing except Sakhalin. *Mania sachalinosa.*'

The need to seek official permission from suspicious admin-istrators was a bug-bear. The unctuous Galkin-Vraskoy, head of the Prison Services, while apparently giving the go-ahead, actually circulated a memo to his regional directors forbidding Chekhov access to the political prisoners. Suvorin, on the other hand, clearly a forerunner of the twentieth-century newspaper magnate in his attitude to officialdom, ignored the political sensitivity of the mission and despite his quite reasonable personal misgivings about the whole venture gave Chekhov a press card and the financial resources needed to complete his journey. Chekhov's method of repaying Suvorin was to send sketches to Moscow from his over-land journey east of Tyumen, across the Yenisey to Irkutsk and the last stretch along the Amur River to Nicolayevsk; these were published in instalments in *New Times* as they were written.

His association with Suvorin had always aroused fierce jealousy on the part of Chekhov's contemporaries, who accused him of being Suvorin's 'kept woman'. No one ever accused Chekhov of being politically small-minded, but *New Times* was an instru-ment of reaction; and for some of his contemporaries—the liberal reformer and engineer Garin-Mikhailovsky, for one—Suvorin was the devil incarnate. Chekhov was astute about people. Accused of being 'unprincipled' by an editor, he replied: 'I have never toadied, nor lied, nor insulted.' Nor, he added for good measure, had he ever written a line he was ashamed of. Though several of his family found employment thanks to Suvorin, he never allowed this debt to impinge on his freedom to speak his mind. Their letters are frank, and reveal a more outspoken man than the rather respectable writer cultivated by three generations of Soviet censors; at times Chekhov is bawdy, and even frankly misogynistic. Politically, he and Suvorin agreed about almost nothing in their letters, and were poles apart temperamentally—yet their relationship lasted until the dispute that fanned across Europe in the wake of Zola's intervention in the Dreyfus affair.

Chekhov almost managed to convince his close friend, the painter Isaak Levitan, to accompany him at least part of the way to Siberia. Levitan finally backed out, saying that he didn't want to abandon his mistress for such a long time. He was a landscape painter who liked to include elements of social history in his work: one of his widescreen paintings, *Vladimirka* (1892), depicts the bare dirt track on which so many convicts died on their way into exile. Chekhov was no less an enthusiast of the steppe: ever since his childhood in Taganrog, where 'those boundless plains of waving grasses, streams and gullies' started on the far side of the cemetery, it had represented freedom for him.

What is most noticeable about Levitan's painting, however, is that the giant outdoors itself is a kind of prison.

The nine instalments Chekhov wrote for Suvorin's paper and posted back to Moscow from Tomsk, Irkutsk and the Baikal region (they are collected under the title *Across Siberia*) are breezy travel sketches. Chekhov recounts how his horse-driven tarantass, an uncomfortable springless carriage, came within a hair's breadth of colliding with three post troikas racing in the opposite direction, drivers asleep at the reins. Thomas de Quincey's giddy exercises in divagation come to mind: 'We heard our speed, we saw it, we felt it as thrilling; and this speed was not the product of blind insensate agencies, that had no sympathy to give, but was incarnated in the fiery eyeballs of the noblest among brutes, in his dilated nostril, spasmodic muscles, and thunder-beating hoofs.'

Siberia, no less than Sakhalin, was less a physical place than an imaginary topos for most Russians, and Chekhov takes an almost perverse delight in stressing its humdrum qualities, the bandits and wild animals conspicuously absent, his revolver unneeded. Floods and ferries slowed his progress. Once he had to wait fifteen hours before his tarantass could be repaired. Boredom, not fear, seems the taiga's prevailing quality: 'The Siberian Highway is the longest, and I should think, the ugliest road on earth.' But there are expansive moments too: 'The power and enchantment of the taiga lie not in titanic trees or the silence of the graveyard, but in the fact that only birds of passage know where it ends.' The Yenisey River, he thought, was a 'mighty, raging Hercules'.

The high point of the journey seems to have been the last stretch: a thousand miles by steamer on the river Amur to Nikolaievsk on the Pacific coast. As if to confound his own intention of demystifying Sakhalin, he notices that the captain of the boat, *The Baikal*, taking him over the Tatar Strait to the Alexandrovsk, the island's main port, 'does not trust the official charts and follows his own, which he draws up and corrects while sailing'.

Perhaps the captain had been supplied with one of the maps in Jonathan Swift's *Travels into Several Remote Nations of the World*, which advertises a group of strangely named islands in the north Pacific between the coasts of Japan and California. The legend of Belovode, a kind of divine realm located in an archipelago at the edge of the known world, persisted in Russian religious memory until well into the twentieth century: it periodically attracted the attentions of members of a sect called The Wanderers, and of parties of religiously-inspired peasants.

A distant bush fire makes Chekhov's first impressions of the island sound quite ominous: 'I could not see the wharf and buildings through the darkness and the smoke drifting across the sea, and could barely distinguish the dim lights at the post, two of which were red. The horrifying scene was compounded of darkness, silhouettes of mountains, and beyond the mountains, a red glow which rose to the sky, from remote fires. It seemed that all of Sakhalin was in flames.' We were wanderers on prehistoric earth: this is the tone of Marlow's slow symphony of eeriness as he penetrates further and further into the heart of darkness.

If Chekhov is crossing over into a territory that is also a place of the mind, it is not a landscape out of Dante or one of Swift's previsions of a totalitarian society, but something like the heath in a Shakespeare play, that unpatrolled tract of land beyond the city walls where not even a wandering Cynic philosopher would venture. Convicts are bare men living on the floor of basic need. Abject, badly clothed, foul-smelling, they are poor Toms. At this level their needs are animal. Chekhov seems to be pursuing the question that humbles Lear when he loses his crown: what is natural man? What is a human being anyway, outside the walls of the city?

When he disembarked on 9 July 1890, having left Moscow on 21 April, Chekhov found that his visit coincided with the quinquennial visit of the Governor of Eastern Siberia. He also had the luck to meet a junior doctor at the hospital who was a fierce critic of the administration. 'I'm glad you're staying with our enemy,' the island commandant remarked to him, 'now you'll learn about all our little shortcomings.' Then he set to work.

Where a present-day epidemiologist would save his feet by using applied statistical techniques on representative subgroups, Chekhov had ten thousand index cards printed in the local police sweat-shop. He had come like the biblical census-taker. Each card comprised entries for legal status—convict, settled-exile (those who had completed their prison term but had to remain on the island), and peasants-in-exile (who could leave Sakhalin but had to remain in Siberia)—and items for surname, patronymic, settlement, age, religious persuasion, occupation and married status. Diseases were recorded; diet and financial support; the mortality rate. *Why* they had been convicted was not his concern.

Seven-and-a-half thousand of these cards can still be consulted in the Chekhov Archives in Moscow.

For the next few months, he went from shack to barracks and on to the next settlement accompanied by a single guard who carried his inkstand and warned the householders of his imminent arrival. 'The people who live there are a tattered and famished bunch of Russian, Polish, Finnish, Georgian rogues, thrown together by chance, like the survivors of a shipwreck.' Most of the settlements were scattered along the river Tym, and in the western and southern parts of the island; by September 10, having visited all the settlements in the north, Chekhov joined *The Baikal* to sail down to Korsakov, the main town in the milder south.

His work schedule was gruelling, starting at five in the morning and continuing until late at night. He wrote to Suvorin that when he went to bed he was in a state of extreme tension, haunted by what still remained to be done. When he wasn't gathering information he was busy studying the prison records, or drawing up an inventory of equipment lacking in the hospitals. He appears to have enjoyed *carte blanche* from the Governor General, who asked Chekhov to pay a visit: they hit it off, which was just as well, since Galkin-Vraskoy hadn't bothered to inform him that a troublesome writer was on his way.

Only the political prisoners, a mere forty out of the island's population of ten thousand, were out of bounds to Chekhov, a fact which irked him but didn't stand in the way of his main objective: to document the island's penal conditions. At the end of his stay, he was able to say, with only slight exaggeration, that 'there is not a single convict or settled-exile on Sakhalin who hasn't had a chat with me'. Many of them continued to correspond with him long after his departure.

Writing it all up proved more difficult, indeed turned out to be his own ball-and-chain; which must have baffled him, since his apprentice work had itself been a concession to the documentary. He warns a friend his report will be 'tedious, specialised, and consist of nothing but figures': in fact, the few statistics in his book seem largely incidental to the burden of a narrative which keeps the reader, like the obliging inkstand carrier, fully in view. Vladimir Nabokov once remarked that Chekhov had a poor dictionary and only a few verbal effects, yet managed to be one of the most subtle writers.

Chekhov was appalled that lip service should be paid to reform, while actual conditions showed up the blatant lack of interest in 'civilising' the prisoners. Some prisoners were assigned to fell and lug timber, a gruelling occupation which exposed them, because they were shackled to the logs, to the risk of freezing to death.

How were these men to become good householders on completing their prison terms, he wondered, if the brutalising conditions of their prison sentence forced them to abandon any domestic habits they had acquired in their earlier life?

More than once he mocks himself as the 'write-write man' (as the indigenous Galyaks call him): disembarking at the pier he noted that 'all 50 [convicts] took off their caps—very likely no such honour has ever been accorded a single literary figure to this day'. Reasonable, unruffled, not put out by circumstances—Chekhov's journey might hint at his wish to earn the right to mock himself 'doing time'.

That impression should not go unchallenged. Our conviction that life lived at the extremes is somehow more authentic than ordinary life (a revival of Hobbes' belief in mortal danger as the ideal condition for self-knowledge) wouldn't have been Chekhov's. 'Only in the settlers' barracks near the mine and here in Derbinskoye, on that raining, muddy morning,' he wrote in this abyss of neglect, 'did I live through moments when I felt that I saw before me the extreme limits of man's degradation.'

The moral lesson of human life lived at the zoological level—Lear's lesson—is dreadfully simple: it has none to offer. It isn't sympathy and respect that attend the spectacle of natural man, but revulsion. Natural man is the shame of nature.

For all that he attempted to suppress subjective turns, a lyric surge is never far from the lull of Chekhov's prose. His descriptions of the kale-gatherers on the coast and the simple funeral ceremony in Alexandrovsk where the gravediggers talk 'about some business of their own' and a recently bereaved orphan laughs grotesquely at his mother's graveside reveal him trying to suppress his own narrative gift.

Soon after his arrival, for example, he visits the Alexandrovsk hard-labour prison, reserved mostly for prisoners who had done a runner from the island across Siberia. In winter they could escape over the pack ice that joined Sakhalin to the mainland, and risk frostbite and death by exposure; in summer they had to stow away on a boat. It seems an utterly desperate act; Chekhov estimates that two out of three prisoners had tried to escape at one time or another. Hope, as the Russian proverb goes, is always last to die. Most would be recaptured within a few weeks, or perish in the wilds. Those who were recaptured got the lash. In his history of Australia's settlement, *The Fatal Shore* (1986), Robert Hughes mentions that whenever the early Botany Bay convicts escaped inland they often headed north, thinking they would come eventually to 'China': the geographic sense of prisoners on Sakhalin was probably no more acute.

Yet even in such dingy, stunted circumstances Chekhov's lists are exuberant with ordinariness, with what the British Empire's version of *deportatio in insulam* called bags and iron: 'On the boards lie caps, boots, bits of bread, empty milk bottles stopped up with a bit of paper or old rag, and shoe-trees; under the boards are chests, filthy sacks, bundles, tools and various bits of old clothing [...] On the walls hang clothes, pots and tools, and on the shelves are teapots, loaves and boxes of something or other.'

Further down the west coast, in Dooay—'a dreadful, hideous place, wretched in every respect, in which only saints or profoundly perverse people could live of their own free will'—hardened prisoners were chained to wheelbarrows. The company of five men in St Petersburg who ran the mines, he notes, was guaranteed an annual profit of 150,000 roubles.

For all Chekhov's evident disgust at the kulakism of its coal-quarries, the moral censure and sensationalism that stalk so many contemporary Victorian philanthropic reports on urban living conditions are quite alien to his approach. 'Their crimes', he remarks, looking at these supposedly hardened recidivists, 'were no more clever and cunning than their faces'.

Even unspeakable places can become home. Walking down Main Street with him, it is hardly the penal reformer we hear:

It is always quiet in Dooay. The ear soon grows accustomed to the slow, measured jangling of the fetters, the thunder of the breakers on the sea and the humming of telegraph wires, and because of these sounds the impression of dead silence grows still stronger. Severity and rigorousness lie imprinted not merely on the striped posts. If somebody should unexpectedly burst into loud laughter in the street, it would sound harsh and unnatural. Life here has taken on a form which can be communicated only through hopeless and implacably cruel sounds, and the ferocious cold wind which on winter nights blows in the cleft from the sea is the only thing which sings precisely the right note.

Chekhov's interest in other people's lives never flags. Underlining the island's parodic relationship to metropolitan Russia, he lists the convicts' adopted or acquired names: Ivan don't-remember-my-name and Man-whose-title-no-one-knows, or epithets like the names of the devils in Dante's hell: Limper, Stomach, Godless, Bone-idle. Gogol has names like those too, in *Dead Souls*.

These epic names are followed by an exploded-view drawing of the Russian water closet and the theory of 'reverse draught'. To his disgust there was no latrine at all at Kosov, where the prisoners were led out in groups to relieve themselves on the street. His descriptions of giant burdocks and umbellates in Novo-Mikhailovka are lengthy and botanically exact. On one occasion, straying into Dostoevskian territory, his account of the flogging of a vagabond called Prokhorov contrasts fascinatingly with the other writer's sensationalism, and is chilling in its spareness:

'Prokhorov does not utter a single word, but simply bellows and wheezes; it seems as if, since the punishment began, a whole eternity has passed, but the overseer is calling only: "Forty-*two*! Forty-*three*!" There is a long way to go to ninety. I walk outside.'

Most other writers would have lingered on the voyeuristic scope of an incident like that—not Chekhov. This is a foretaste of the mature writer who has learned that less is more. Chekhov's intention to immerse us, and himself, in the grittiness of life on Sakhalin fails him completely at one point in the book. The fact-gatherer gets his pockets picked, as it were, by the lyric dramatist. An unexpected safari view of the island rears out of the dark on an evening drive above Alexandrovsk: 'the gigantic burdock leaves seemed like tropical plants, while the dark hills loomed in on all sides. Away in the distance were fires where people were burning coal, and there would be a light from a forest fire. The moon would rise. Suddenly, a fantastic picture: trundling to meet us along the rails, on a small platform, a convict leaning on a pole, dressed all in white.'

This passage escaped the revisions of what he called his 'purple patches'; it is one which gets close to the heart of what makes *A Journey to Sakhalin* so compelling.

Expanding his comments on Chekhov's language, Nabokov wrote that he 'keeps all his words in the same dim light and of the same exact tint of grey, a tint between the colour of an old fence and that of a low cloud'. Low-wattage moments of odd intensity are to be found in the mature œuvre too, mingled with a weight of felt experience that is all the more painfully vivid for its drab and formless surroundings: at the close of *Ward No. 6*, on the afternoon after being beaten up, Dr Ragin grasps that he is dying: suddenly he sees dart past in the gathering dark, 'a herd of deer, extraordinarily handsome and graceful, of which he had been reading on the previous day'. His consciousness does not end there. 'A peasant woman stretched out her hand to him with a registered letter.' But its contents are not revealed, either to us or to Dr Ragin.

'You need equanimity in this world', Chekhov told Suvorin, 'only people with equanimity can see things clearly, be fair and work'. Work is what Conrad's Marlow calls 'efficiency', the device for getting through a life with dignity. Chekhov's insight—part-social, part-psychological—into that 'grey, ordinary' life was to see it as a kind of bookkeeping that never really adds up. 'You confuse two things,' he wrote to Suvorin, '*solving* a problem and *stating* a problem *correctly*. It is only the second that is obligatory for the artist.'

Yet literature must have form, even a literature of loose ends. Like Turgenev, Chekhov understood that life has its own forms of being, and that they are more complex than our schemes for understanding them—'for all things in nature influence one another, and even the fact that I have just sneezed is not without its influence on surrounding nature'. This was the attentive contemporary of Henri Poincaré whose famous article in *Acta Mathematica* in 1889 anticipated what is now called chaos theory; Chekhov himself asserted often enough that his medical training had moulded him as a writer. It is surprising that so few critics have taken him at his word, though one who did, the philosopher Lev Shestov, accused him of 'killing human hopes'.

Randomness and contingency are major forces in Chekhov's

art, in its almost brutal lack of sentimentality: the great crisis of Victorian theism was already behind him—he saw no compelling reason to deny the existence of God because he never saw any overriding reason to affirm it. As he told Suvorin, a writer should know better than to speculate about the existence of God. It was left to Tolstoy, the involuntary egoist, to wonder what humans might be if only they could realise their essential nature in the light of the Sermon on the Mount; Chekhov remained an unworried child of Hume. It would be wrong to suggest that he was a man without faith: Russia without faith would be unendurable. Work was the answer.

His attitude to life can best be described as a distrust of attitudes to life; it is surely scepticism that bestows upon him his equanimity and wry amusement, and general lack of resentment about the doings of time. To put it another way: if Tolstoy saw the lie, Chekhov saw what seeing the lie occluded.

Chekhov returned from 'hell' on October 13, sailing on the liner *St Petersburg*, which called in at Vladivostock, Hong Kong ('a glorious bay'), Ceylon ('a heavenly place') and the Suez Canal; he travelled with two mongooses, a palm civet and a hairless Buryat priest. All were to lodge with him in his Moscow flat for varying lengths of time, and the mongoose eventually became quite domesticated, if something of an annoyance for the friends who stopped by to visit him in his flat in formal clothes—it liked to chew hats.

After recovering from a deterioration in his general condition over the winter, he began work towards publication of his Sakhalin book in his 'out-of-surgery' hours, on Mondays, Tuesdays and Wednesdays, a period in which he combined clinical work on his own estate at Melikhovo with civic duties as an unpaid medical inspector during an outbreak of cholera. Guests and family harried him for all sorts of favours, and often he had to stonewall them to secure time for writing.

The year after Sakhalin he went on a grand tour of some of the great European cities, including Vienna and Venice, and took in their opulence and architecture with the same fascination he had shown, under rather different conditions, for the people of Siberia.

Being a prison island inspector was just one of Chekhov's many parallel lives; in those years he even tried to set up a scheme to rescue a financially ailing journal of surgery.

Relatively few stories emerged from his Siberian trip—*Gusev*, *In Exile*, *The Murder* (which, in its four pages, does what he couldn't achieve in his report's three hundred pages, according to Janet Malcolm) and *Peasant Woman*—as though insisting to his detractors, who had accused him of going in search of novelty, how serious he was about his objectives. His was to be a book outside the charmed codex of literature.

When *Journey to Sakhalin* appeared three years later, some of it having been serialised by the journal *Russian Thought*, the Russian delegate at the Fifth World Prison Congress in Paris had to answer repeated questions about carceral conditions on the island. The notoriety of the American reporter George Kennan's investigation *Siberia and the Exile System*, published in New York in 1891, had fanned the interest. Perhaps his own book didn't achieve everything Chekhov had hoped of it, but its publication certainly dispelled the utopian fantasy of transforming Sakhalin into an agricultural colony. The extended passage in his book that describes the lashing of the unfortunate Prokhorov caused a public outcry. A government commission was sent to investigate prisoners' conditions on the island in 1896; and corporal punishment of women was abolished the following year (and of men in 1904). Chekhov himself organised a dispatch of thousands of books for use in the local schools. On 2 January 1894, finished with his corrections, he wrote to Suvorin:

'Medicine can no longer reproach me with being unfaithful: I've paid a proper tribute to erudition, and to what old writers call pedantry. And I'm happy that a convict's rough smock is hanging in my literary wardrobe too. Let it hang there!'

Journey to Sakhalin is a work of a quite different order from the *The Seagull* or *The Cherry Orchard* or any of the marvellous stories, but it deserves a place alongside them, rather than being consigned to the mere paragraph it gets in some biographies (William Gerhardi's, for instance): it is Chekhov's most militantly hopeful book. It is also by far his longest work. He was protesting against injustice in his own way—a writer who happened to be a doctor, whose formative training had been in the empirical methods of the natural sciences.

Chekhov never doubted individuals could make a difference. Pages are blank like tundra, and freedom is our ability to surprise ourselves by leaving a mark on them. The essayist Hubert Butler once observed of Chekhov's individualism that 'his faith is so soberly expressed as to be proof against all disillusionment.' It is a sound observation. In his desire to civilise Russia by modest improvements—he once accused the Moscow intellectuals of being blinded by their grand utopian schemes and scientifically organised dreams of society to the real achievements of the *zemstva*, those local government bodies set up in the 1860s to build hospitals and other civic amenities (and which in the last days of tsardom employed that other brilliant doctor-writer Mikhail Bulgakov)—his visit to Sakhalin looks like an excursion to a century that will be remembered not just for its material improvements but for revealing what utopia means: internment camps and total surveillance. When Humanity becomes a perfect transcendent unity, humans don't just lose their civic status and end up as poor Toms—they become superfluous. The twentieth century showed beyond doubt that philanthropy, as Edmund Burke suggested in one of his pungent asides, has homicidal tendencies too.

Perhaps Chekhov's visit to the prison colony at the back gates of Russia explains why his theatre sets seem so empty, abandoned to the implicating dimension of time—recalled a dozen times at the opening of *Three Sisters*—and the shelter of an enclosed garden extending into the wings, out of our field of vision. Moonlight glints on the shards of bottle-glass strewn along the crest of the wall. 'If only we could know', Olga's cry concludes that play, 'oh if only we could know'.

Sakhalin stands in the same haunting relationship to Chekhov's literary work as the darker meanings that hover over the garden wall.

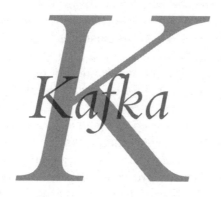

Uncle Siegfried

SCENES FROM A WORLD OF TRUST
INFECTED BY SUSPICION

Large print

After working for a year as a country doctor in Scotland, I came across a slim pale-green hardback in Hugendubel's sixties-style bookshop overlooking the Marienplatz in Munich, and read it through my first winter away. It was a bibliophile edition of Franz Kafka's *Ein Landarzt* (*A Country Doctor*) published by the small Berlin press run by Klaus Wagenbach, himself one of Kafka's biographers, to celebrate thirty years in the book business.

The history of the book is a striking reminder that Kafka's fame as a writer was not entirely posthumous. Written mostly in his sister Ottla's apartment in the famous medieval Alchemists' Lane in Prague as 'the war to end all wars' turned to disaster for the Dual Empire of Austro-Hungary, *Ein Landarzt* appeared in January 1920, and received a single notice in the *Prager Tagblatt* newspaper months after publication. Of the 1000 copies printed in outsize Tertia Walbaum typeface, few—very few—were purchased in Kafka's lifetime (the other six books he published were also flops). The publishing house of Schocken Verlag, subsequently to relocate to New York, took over the unsold remainder copies in the 1930s.

Like the original, this new edition of the stories is printed in the large typeface opted for by Kafka's original publisher; it was so large in the Walbaum Antiqua typeface of the first edition that hyphens had to be halved and punctuation marks omitted to fit the line. Kafka's early writings—which often expand a single seamless paragraph into an entire story—are sometimes so brief as to impose the large format and spacious margins, not least if his publisher needed a book that could be marketed. That his few thoughts had acquired such lapidary scale was a source of occasional embarrassment: Kafka was reminded of Moses and the Ten Commandments.

A final bibliographic connection: this new edition is printed by the Offizin Haag-Drugulin in Leipzig, one of the most famous printers in Germany and the same house that produced *The Penal Colony* for Kafka's original publisher Kurt Wolff.

Another genealogy

Kafka dedicated his book to his father. According to his friend Max Brod, his father is supposed to have muttered 'put it on the table by my bed'; Hermann Kafka's refusal to acknowledge his son's literary activities is hardly one of the secrets of a well-documented fraught relationship. But the title figure of the collection— the country doctor—honours a different relative altogether, his uncle.

Siegfried Löwy was born in 1867, elder half-brother to Kafka's mother and, following his MD at the University of Prague, possessor of the only doctorate in the family until his nephew's, although many of Kafka's mother's family harboured scholastic, even talmudic ambitions. Significantly, Franz often thought of himself as a Löwy rather than a Kafka: his diary entry for 25 December 1911 contains a long list of colourful matrilineal *begats*, including a reference to his maternal great-grandfather, who was a miracle rabbi. 'In Hebrew my name is Amschel, like my mother's maternal grandfather, whom my mother, who was six years old when he died, can remember as a very pious and learned man with a long, white beard. She remembers how she had to take hold of the toes of his corpse and ask forgiveness for any offence she might have committed against him. She also remembers his many books, which lined the walls. He bathed in the river every day, even in winter, when he chopped a hole in the ice for his bath.'

In his famous *Letter to His Father* he defined himself as 'a Löwy with a certain Kafka component which, however, is not pushed ahead by the Kafka will to life, business and conquest, but by a Löwyish spur that works more secretly, more diffidently and in another direction, and which often fails to work entirely'. One of the Löwyish spurs was his TB, which he tended to describe as if it were a conspiracy of organs: 'Sometimes, it seems to me that my brain and lungs came to an agreement behind my back. Things can't go on this way, said the brain, and after five years the lungs said they were ready to help.' Even the unpleasant transformation of the travelling salesman Gregor Samsa, in Kafka's most famous story *Metamorphosis*, into a hundred-footed insect covered with 'sticky stuff' seems morphologically related to Kafka's tuberculosis: the repulsive appearance of the insect (which assures his victimisation) is in fact an *inside*: an eventrated respiratory tract replete with cilia and mucus carpet.

A doctor of law he might have been in life, but Kafka's real doctorate was handed down by an imaginary guild, the Faculty of Concepts to Live and Die By. Despite Koch's demonstration of the bacillary nature of tuberculosis in 1882, Kafka always interpreted his illness as a metaphor: what power could a bare fact have against a death sentence issued at birth?

An early speedster

While his nephew was in his last years at school, Uncle Siegfried took up a post in Triesch, a small town of 4800 inhabitants in a German-speaking enclave in Moravia called Iglau (known in Czech as Jihlava), about 130 kilometres south-east of Prague. Nearly half the local population was of German origin, and it boasted several small industries including wool and spinning factories, and a mineworks. He was to practise there for close on forty years.

Siegfried Löwy was a liberal (he almost *had* to be as a university-educated assimilated Jew) and man of his times; open to change and innovation, he created a sensation in the district when he became one of the first people in what was then an outpost of the Austro-Hungarian Empire to acquire a motorbike. Franz came visiting many times in his summer holidays, the great attractions of staying with Uncle Siegfried being his horses, the billiard table and the library, which contained all the German classics. There were also the mechanical appliances—a photograph in the book shows his nieces, including Kafka's sister Ottla, push-starting Uncle Siegfried on his brand-new bike across a forest path.

According to Hans Straße, Head Conservationist of the Motorcycle Department of the Deutsches Museum in Munich, the tin panniers behind the seat and the distinctive rear shock absorbers identify it as a NSU Cantilever, built in Ulm between 1909 and 1914: NSU (later amalgamated in the Audi concern) was one of more than fifty motorcycle manufacturers in the Europe of that time. Since the world speed record was set on this machine in 1909, it may well be that Kafka's uncle, a 'munterer Vogel' (an oddball) as he might have called himself, read about the exploit and ordered a model for his practice rounds. Improved transportation was changing the nature of the medical profession, and speed would come to alter the very shape of the consultation. Doctors were among the first enthusiasts of vehicular transport, but most of them bought the rather stately sedans and berlins of the period. Dr Löwy's speedster motorbike would no doubt have amused the wags in Triesch.

Holisms

Unlike Kafka's father, the self-made man, Uncle Siegfried indulged Franz, and offered him advice and support at several junctures in his life. He was 'progressive' in his medical thinking too. On his recommendation Franz became a vegetarian, and for a time practised the obscure double-chewing technique ('each mouthful to be masticated thirty-two times') recommended by the American physician Horace Fletcher (1849–1919) along with Johannes Müller's free air gymnastic techniques (developing the body was a cult, of course, long before the Nazis made it a key element of their cultural propaganda).

'Fletschern' and 'müllern', as they were rather rudely described, were the alternative therapies of the early twentieth century, and the physically slight Kafka seems to have hoped that such regular cud-chewing and callisthenics would deflect his conviction that his illness was prefigured, not just historically, but in a primordial sense—as if it were inscribed on his body. 'My body is too skinny for its weakness, it hasn't the least bit of fat to produce a blessed warmth, to preserve an inner fire, no fat on which the spirit could occasionally nourish itself beyond its daily need without damage to the whole.'

Uncle and nephew both travelled together to the German North Sea islands of Heligoland and Nordeney after the completion of Franz's school exams. Much later, in February 1924, in the last months of his nephew's life, when he was living a *vie de bohème* in Berlin with a young Jewish girl from the eastern marches called Dora Dymant (or Dora Diamant, as she called herself after she emigrated to Britain before the war), his uncle visited him and persuaded him to enter a sanatorium. This was the happiest period of Kafka's life, according to Brod; it is known that Kafka wrote to Dora's Yiddish-speaking orthodox father asking for permission to marry her: the rabbi prudently said no. Brod was a tireless friend: he even arranged the visit from Uncle Siegfried because doctors' fees were proving too expensive: Dora mentions having to pay 160 crowns for a house visit at a time when all they had to pay the rent and buy provisions was Kafka's invalidity pension of one thousand crowns a month.

Siegfried Löwy continued to practise in his house in Triesch until his retirement in the mid-thirties, when he moved to Prague and set up residence together with his nieces—the Kafka sisters, Elli, Valli and Ottla—and their families, in the large house in the Bilkova left by Hermann, Franz's father. The night before the extended family was due to be deported to the death-camps in 1942, Siegfried Löwy drew up his will and injected himself with a lethal dose of morphine.

Semi-colons

His nephew's story A Country Doctor seems to be goaded on by its semicolons.

According to the literary critic Walter Benjamin, who recorded their conversations in Sweden while both were on the run from the Nazis in 1934, the dramatist Bertolt Brecht, famous in his lifetime for his agitprop theatre and Communist ideals, accused Kafka of having the 'precision of an imprecise man: a dreamer'; it is apparent from *A Country Doctor* how Brecht could formulate such a dismissive statement, even if he does resort to Kafkaesque method to do so. Kafka uses one of the simplest grammatical markings to set up several layers of apparently banal realism in which quite bizarre things happen without fuss, as matter of fact; his famous sliding paradoxes actually begin at the level of parasyntactic notation, at what are usually termed the accidentals.

The first sentence announces: 'I was at my wits' end: an urgent journey lay before me'. A colon buffers the adjoining phrases, in which five semicolons marshall the subordinate clauses into separate stretches of time and action and necessity. The American writer Nicholson Baker has called the semi-colon 'that supremely self-possessed valet of phraseology'; and the literary critic Erich Heller once drew attention to a 'profound' semicolon in a remark by the philosopher Wittgenstein: 'The philosopher treats a question; like a disease' where the profundity turns on whether the semicolon ought to play the comma and make questioning itself a kind of disease.

From his manuscripts, we know that Kafka had a fairly idiosyncratic system of notation when entering early versions of his stories in his notebooks. He used commas and periods; semicolons were added only when work was being prepared for publication. (In the case of his novel *The Trial*, they were added posthumously by his friend Max Brod, to whom he had given the loose manuscript.) But perhaps we should regard the semicolon more conspiratorially than Baker's 'valet status' would suggest: commenting on his friend Isaac Babel's laconic stories, Sergei Eisenstein, the great Russian film director, said—speaking of what literature could teach the cinema—'no iron can enter the human heart with such stupefying effect as a period placed at just the right moment'.

If periods are bullets, then Kafka's semicolons are spurs. They edge one phrase recklessly on to the next, and barely hold them all in check. They wink at the doctor's cognitive disarray—he is hardly through taking the measure of one set of circumstances before another falls upon him.

Only a doctor

It all starts with the narrator, the country doctor, at wit's end—'in a dwam', as some of my Scottish country patients would have said. A reportedly ill patient is awaiting his visit in a village ten miles off. He bemoans his lack of transport, his own horse having just died in the terrible winter weather. 'But you just don't know what you're going to stumble across in your own house', says the servant girl.

In the shortest possible grammatical time, the doctor has come across a groom, two horses which squeeze through the keyhole (from a pig-sty, a buried reference to the treatment reserved for the string of horses in the novella *Michael Kohlhaas* by the nineteenth-century German writer Heinrich von Kleist), abandoned his maid to the groom's cannibalistic designs on her (he bites her cheek), and arrived through a snowstorm in a flash at his patient's bed. Demons have been unleashed. These can only be Mephistopheles' horses, on loan from Goethe's *Faust*. The miraculous transport is itself described in a sentence with no less than eleven semicolons. It is a breakneck, lightning-speed journey that has a precedent in some of the Hasidic stories: Kafka would have known these from the famous collection published by the philosopher Martin Buber, in which the Ba'al Shem-tov (the honorary title of Rabbi Israel ben Eli'ezer, c. 1700–1760, the founder of Hasidism) is summoned to perform wonder cures at the drop of a hat. The Yiddish writer Isaac Bashevis Singer's later stories are full of such dropped hats.

For Kafka's doctor, however, any idea of a wonder cure is sheer parody. Already the patient is whispering into his ear, 'Let me die.' At first glance there's nothing wrong with him; as the doctor gets ready to leave he notices a huge wound on the right side near the hip seething with what look like larval forms of the common house fly *Musca domestica*. Another tradition—the Greek, in the story of Endymion and Selene—tells us the fly was once a beautiful, if excessively talkative girl; and since so many other half-hidden things are happening in this story, we could be forgiven for assuming the patient laid low by the seeds of love. After all, in Shakespeare's time love was still considered an 'illness' (*morbus amoris*).

Some critics have thought the wound an act of self-castration or self-division, like the wound that won't heal in *Parsifal*, although it would seem more obviously related to the place where Adam, before God closed it again, might have had his fatal rib extraction; in any case it is difficult to miss the equation of the maid Rose and the horribly pink gap in the skin—the wound recalls the supposedly ancient male fear of the female genitals. Kafka, with his keen instinct for ambiguities, is confusing the absolute distinction that medical ethics tries to maintain between the roles of doctor and lover: this is a prerequisite to the art of effective diagnosis. Besides, remembering Rose during the consultation is a sure sign that the country doctor's mind isn't entirely engaged with the nature of his patient's complaint.

'Will you save me?', pleads the patient, having evidently changed his mind. Under his breath, the doctor berates the community for its loss of belief; people are always expecting the impossible from the doctor's healing hand. This is a community of our time, which 'no longer believes in God', as Nietzsche wrote in one of his extended aphorisms, though 'there are still plenty of thinking people who believe in the saint'. The country doctor is indeed a kind of 'saint'—an ascetic, self-denying figure in a material age—of whom miracles are expected.

Then a posse of villager elders arrives at the house with the school choir and teacher at its head, and sings a simple song denouncing doctors:

Strip him naked, then he'll heal us
And should he fail to, kill him quick!
Only a mediciner, only a mediciner.

A saint is expected, but only a doctor turns up—a mediciner, a saw-bones. The country doctor is human, all too human, the title Nietzsche gave to the book in which he examined what might make for saintliness in an age of unbelief. Stripped of his clothes, the villagers lift him head and feet onto the bed, 'on the side of the wound'. His patient complains he's always had to grin and put up with things, and doesn't appreciate having to share his bed; the doctor consoles him with false reassurance: such wounds aren't uncommon in the wider world. And anyway, it seems to be a case of Munchhausen's syndrome, a couple of self-mutilating blows with the blade of an axe. Self-knowledge was never easier; but there's no cure for the wound that comes from the struggle between reality and reason.

Menaced, outmanoeuvred, and threatened by the massed ranks of the community, the hapless country doctor bears more than a passing resemblance to the epithet-title for the honest man in Henrik Ibsen's suggestively named drama *An Enemy of the People*. Effect and cause are disjoined in much the same way as the doctor who fails his test of saintliness, revealing ordinary human vulnerability: Gregor Samsa's offence, in *Metamorphosis*, is even less an operation of the will—he merely has to wake up to find he *is* what he dreamed he was. The country doctor's fear that he may be 'misused for sacred purposes' is not entirely groundless: all persecutors attribute to their victims the capacity to do harm as well as its reverse. Then he catches himself: 'But now it was time for me to think of saving myself.'

He runs from them, the children chanting a new song behind him: 'Now be cheerful, all you patients, Doctor's laid in bed beside you!' In contrast to his coming, his going is sluggish. Fleeing his patients, unsure whether he'll get back home, his maid seized by the groom, his shaman's fur coat out of reach, cast out into an Arctic desert whose contours are similar to those glimpsed at the conclusion of one of Kafka's eeriest one-page stories 'The Bucket Rider' (the final phrase of which reads: 'And with that I ascend into the regions of the ice mountains and am lost never to be seen again'), the doctor's closing words are no less extraordinary than the entire story: 'Betrayed! Betrayed! Respond to a false alarm on the night bell—and it can't be made good, ever again.'

Despite doing his duty, morally and professionally—indeed striving to fulfil it in sectarian conditions seemingly emptied of the usual ethical-legal content—he ends up stripped of authority, all his clothes and in bed with the patient, and even then might not get home because he has dared upset the natural order (despite trying to shirk off his responsibilities at one point by asserting that he is 'no world reformer'). In doing his duty he has put Rosa, his own hidden wound, out of sight and mind.

One thing remains to be said about the country doctor and his sense of duty: Kafka allows the possibility that his fatal error was to deny his other duty—to himself. The alarm on the night-bell is described as 'false', and in following its bidding he takes an 'Irrweg'—the wrong path. Only near the end does he recollect the life he has been missing; but it is too late. Kafka's story holds up for inspection the Christian view of self-denial as a virtue, and then mocks it as a folly.

This is not Kafka's last word on self-denial.

Medical euphemisms

As Erich Heller observed regarding that same quote by Wittgenstein, a semicolon may sometimes mark the frontier between a thought and a triviality.

Kafka offers us a pathetic sight, a parody of uprightness: a doctor stripped bare by his patients, even. 'Certainly doctors are stupid, or rather, they're not more stupid than other people but their pretensions are ridiculous; nonetheless you have to reckon with the fact that they become more and more stupid the moment you come into their clutches...', he informs Milena Jesenská early on in their correspondence.

His diary entry for 5 March 1912 contains an unflattering portrayal of the kind of bullishly insensitive doctor who, together with his Pooterish judgement on the serving girl (presumably she couldn't afford his full fee), has survived fairly intact into the era of can-do medicine, where he may be more of a menace: 'These revolting doctors! Businesslike, determined and so ignorant of healing that, if this businesslike determination were to leave them, they would stand at sick-beds like schoolboys. I wish I had the strength to found a nature-cure society. By scratching around in my sister's ear Dr K. turns an inflammation of the eardrum into an inflammation of the inner ear; the servant collapses while getting the fire going; with the fleet diagnosis which is his wont in the case of serving staff, the doctor declares it an upset stomach and a resulting congestion of the blood. The next day she takes to her bed again, has a high fever; the doctor turns her from side to side, confirms it is a throat infection, and runs away so that the next moment won't refute him. Even dares to speak of the "vulgarly violent reaction of the girl", which is true to this extent, that he is used to people whose physical condition is worthy of his curative power and is produced by it, and he feels insulted, more than he is aware, by the strong nature of this country girl.'

Kafka mistakenly attributes his sister's ear infection to the 'inner' ear (it should be 'middle'); his judgement on the Hausarzt—'ignorant of healing'—strikes hard. Having consulted more than a few doctors in his time, Kafka was no doubt used to being treated by them as if his body were merely a fleshy appendage to his lungs— those 'proud strong tormented imperturbable creatures'. His diary is peppered with symptoms ('a new headache of a kind unknown so far', 'I had a slight spell of faintness', 'this past week I suffered something like a breakdown') which are watched over with the fastidiousness of a true hypochondriac.

In June 1914, well before he first coughed up blood (which he experienced, significantly, as a kind of relief: 'actually, my headaches seem to have been washed away with the flow of blood'), he had written to Grete Bauer: 'undoubtedly an enormous hypochondria, which however has struck so many and such deep roots within me that I stand or fall with it'. Keenly observant of the theatrical aspects of his uncle's practice, and of the euphemous sounds of doctors in general ('catarrh of the apex of the lungs'), Kafka sets the country doctor up for what doctors routinely subject their patients to but undergo rarely themselves, and then only by peers, as humiliation and primal fear: defrocking.

A plague of doctors

Being familiar with doctors who suffer diseases for their patients in folk stories, how, we might wonder, forgetting that *A Country Doctor* was written in the early days of psychoanalysis, could a doctor suffer a wound for his patient? Is he being punished for his impatience by the spurs of those opening semicolons? Half a century before the French literary critic Michel Foucault deconstructed the power relations of the medical profession, Kafka identifies the surgeon's able hand as dispensing with the need for the confessional, the redundant cleric—in a telling image—sitting down desolately to unravel his raiment. It is an abdication: the cleric embodies the collapse of a religiously-inspired idealism, but his renunciation prepares the way for the fall of the country doctor too. Kafka astutely sees that the Platonic idea of science as the quest for truth is bound to the decline of the transcendental affirmations of religion. Both are acts of faith, and the practical reason of science will also be undermined by the same empiricism that first displaced religion.

Doctor-baiting has long been a clandestinely popular activity in country regions. Despite the onslaught of progress and professionals with black bags it still enjoys a vogue in some parts of the world; my grandmother in Glasgow used to say, 'that's but ae doctor's opinion', meaning that one mere doctor still had a lot to learn about real wisdom. In country areas, where people have long memories, it is still remembered that doctors themselves were once a sort of plague.

As if to confirm her, the recently published writings of David Rorie (1867–1946), an Aberdeenshire doctor and amateur anthropologist who collected folk medical nostrums and maxims in rural Fife and Aberdeen in the first decades of the twentieth century, clearly show that doctors have only ever been one of several possible sources of reassurance in parochial communities, and that the transmission of learning and knowledge often work against the grain of common sense. It is not just a Scottish phenomenon. Indeed, Emanuel Strauss' extraordinary *Dictionary of Proverbs* tells us that every European language has its saws against the saw-bones.

These are some of the variations on Strauss' entry 1582. Latin: 'errores medicorum terra tegit': English: 'physicians' faults are covered with earth'; German: 'junger Arzt, höckriger Kirchhof'; Dutch: 'een nieuw medicijnmeester een nieuw kerkhof'; Danish: 'ny læge—ny kirkegaard'; French: 'de jeune médecin, cimetière bossu'; Czech: 'nedospelý lékar, hotový záhubce'. All of them are variations on an original observation by the ancient Greek poet Nicocles. Rorie tells us the Scots rhyme on this is:

When the doctor cures,
    The sun sees it.
But when he kills,
    The earth hides it.

Writing recipes

I don't know if Uncle Siegfried had to go out on snowy nights to answer a call (surely he did), but the ditties quoted by Kafka in the story seem inspired by his uncle, who was a wisecracker and self-deprecating joker—quite unlike Kafka's father. Kafka described him to his friend Max Brod as the 'twitterer'—'because such an inhumanly thin, bachelor's, birdlike wit comes piping out of his tightened throat, and never abandons him'. The famous lines in the middle of the story—'Writing prescriptions is easy, but otherwise coming to an understanding with people is hard'—have the ring of the horse's mouth, indeed seem to propel the whole story which, on one level, is simply the enactment of a misunderstanding. Since prescription-writing in German is cognate with what cooks do in the kitchen—writing a recipe (*Rezepte schreiben*) being indisputably more art than science—the country doctor's fate seems to depend on the unpredictable nature of the second half of the saying, on the burden he carries to make himself understood. This is clearer in the original, where the reflexive German verb imposes just such a condition on its grammatical subject (*sich verständigen*).

These days doctors 'negotiate' with their patients, just like Kafka's doctor; and contemporary patients can be just as vague about what it was they wanted help with in the first place. What has happened to the power which the law itself confers on individuals to constitute a meaningful social life? Remove the plea for help, and the doctor has no business being where he is. Kafka underdetermines meaning in his stories to such an extent that potential readings multiply alarmingly when the reader, anxious to reach firmer ground, attempts to place the narrative in a context he himself has supplied.

My interpretation would be this. Nothing is harder to touch than the reality of our lives, and Kafka's rider might be: hardest of all for doctors.

Hell for leather

Bizarrely enough (Kafka's skill with syntax and small words has us driving the narrative on without stopping to question its economy of explanation) this story does have anthropological parallels.

In his diaries, the writer Elias Canetti—a very perceptive Kafkol-ogist—records the following observation by the great German explorer Alexander von Humboldt. 'In thirteenth-century Egypt, a mania for eating human flesh raged through all classes; doctors were the favourite prey. If a man was hungry, he feigned illness and sent for a doctor—not to consult him, but to devour him.' This is confirmed with a note from a Baghdad physician's description of his travels and travails in Egypt: 'people used all possible dupes to waylay others or lure them into their homes on false pretenses. Three doctors who visited me later met with this fate...'

True or not, these observations replicate the internal dynamic of Kafka's story very convincingly. Our hero might not be killed, but his nose gets rubbed in the presumption of wanting to help. Kafka often portrayed fools and clownish figures in his writing; they were beasts of meaningful burden for him as much as they were for the philosopher Nietzsche, who once wrote that fools were a disguise for 'desperate, all too certain knowledge'. That would make Kafka's uncle a Shakespearean nuncle. Some of the most famous English cartoons—Hogarth's and Rowlandson's—lampoon doctors in just the terms suggested by Kafka, as buffoons whose very ministrations were a menace to the bodies of their patients. Perhaps folly and care charge hell for leather out of the same stable; and little wonder if in his moment of adversity the diagnostician, clumsy as he is, has no tradition to shelter in. In a letter to Gershom Scholem in 1938, Benjamin wrote, as part of a critique of Brod's queasily sanctifying biography of Kafka: 'This much Kafka was absolutely sure of: first, that someone must be a fool if he is to help; second, that only a fool's help is real help. The only uncertain thing is whether such help can still do a human being any good.'

Trust lost

As in so many of his stories of individuals thwarted by the forms of life they lead in society at large, Kafka himself seemed to weigh criteria for success in a superdimension where language bears a different charge of trust. Famously dissatisfied with his gifts as a writer, he actually confided to his diary, shortly after finishing *A Country Doctor* in September 1917, that he could still derive 'passing satisfaction' from works like this, provided he could continue to write such things at all; and happiness only if he could raise the world into 'the pure, the true and the immutable'. Those are attributes of the absolute, which is where literature cannot go.

The genius of *A Country Doctor*—and it is not a benign one—resides in the fact that Kafka describes, without naming it, one of the most pressing issues of his society, and all the more of our media-manipulated 'risk society': the issue of trust. It is indeed odd that a man like Kafka, who worked in an insurance office, should have thought safeguards scarcely worth the paper they were written on. His little village in the snow is a world of faith abruptly and unaccountably infected by the language of suspicion. The only strongly individuated character in the story, the doctor, is exposed to a witch hunt. Should we be surprised at the tribal, scapegoating logic that pursues him? Perhaps trust is a kind of non-renewable precapitalist resource that, once depleted, can never be replenished. This concern would account for the lurch into cosmic anguish at the end of the story—'and it can't be made good, ever again'.

Every writer since the Enlightenment has been aware of being condemned to work in this atmosphere of suspicion, so mercilessly diagnosed by Nietzsche and Marx: without a craft tradition (loosely defined as the production and supply of articles needed by the community) the artist's search for meaning is painful, inward, and often absurd. Trust for a writer like Kafka is a primal state that can be regained only by an act of will: that is why he wrote, 'nothing is granted to me, everything has to be earned, not only the present and the future, but the past, too'. Or it can be seized by blind obedience; and Kafka's family history shows how ruthlessly a world of will and illusion was exploited by Hitler, whose inversion of the moral order received shamefully wide support from the 'caring' profession: forty-three percent of German doctors joined the Nazi party in 1933. Trust has lost its pristine quality. At the close of Kafka's century it may be that this quality of trust has eroded further, not just in the artist's despair about 'doing art', but in the citizen's sense of the solidity of those 'substantial categories of state, family and destiny'.

Concluding his recent literary study of trust, Gabriel Josipovici provides a warning and a message of hope: 'But what the art and thought of the past two hundred years teaches us is not the lesson the deconstructionists and post-modernists would draw from it, a lesson of our freedom to live as we want, to choose the stories and traditions we want to live by, the lesson of the hopeless entanglement of all culture and language in hidden struggles for power; it is, rather, that it is not possible to exist without trusting, that to walk and talk and, *a fortiori*, to write and paint and compose is only possible because of trust. When we grasp this we grasp too that denying trust is denying life itself as something that has to be lived in time and in the world of others, the world into which we have been born and in which we will die.'

Pain relief

In his last months, Kafka didn't expect much of his own doctors. 'Verbally I don't learn anything definite, since in discussing the tuberculosis [...] everybody drops into a reticent, evasive, glassy-eyed manner of speech', he wrote to a friend from the sanatorium at Hauptstrasse 187, Kierling, near Vienna, in April 1924.

He'd been brought there by his medical student friend Robert Klopstock, appalled at how he had been treated by Professor Hayek, the imperious Ear, Nose and Throat specialist who was also to operate that same year, with nearly disastrous results, on Freud's oral cancer. That month Kafka weighed a mere 43 kilos (for a height of 180 cm). His TB was now extrapulmonary: it had colonised his larynx, which was acutely inflamed, and from there spread to his epiglottis, effectively preventing him from nourishing himself. Coughing and swallowing must have been searingly painful. 'To think that at one time I could simply dare to take a large gulp of water', he wrote on one of the slips of paper he handed to his friends, under doctors' orders to talk as little as possible.

Those same doctors injected phenol into the superior laryngeal nerve in an attempt to provide relief from pain, but the procedure was only partially successful. To his parents he wrote wonderful, affectionate, cheerful letters, published in their original German only a few years ago after their chance discovery by a Prague bookseller. His letters belie any sense of estrangement or grievance. In them he recalls the swimming lessons his father had given him, the beer and sausages after, and he makes no reference to what he had formerly called 'the disgrace of showing myself undressed in public'. This, a letter about drinking beer, when he was literally dying to have a drink of water but couldn't because of the pain in his throat! He wanted, at all costs, to avoid worrying his parents into visiting him. Dora was there all hours, desperate for the slightest hint of an improvement. He corrected the galley proofs of *A Hunger Artist*, which had just arrived from the publishers. One of the several notes he wrote, perhaps a wry reflection on Hayek and his retinue of medical assistants, was collected and published after his death by Klopstock. It read: 'So the help goes away again without helping.'

To the end, Kafka retained his lucidity; and he left us one of the darkest and funniest Jewish doctor jokes: 'Kill me,' he instructed Klopstock, with whom he had arranged long in advance for a dose of morphine when nothing else availed, 'or else you're a murderer.'

Antinomies

Many of Kafka's stories are explicitly concerned with the individual's relationship to the community (*The Investigations of a Dog*; *The Chinese Wall*; *Josephine, the Singer*); the enthusiasm he spasmodically feels for communal life, like his response to the troupe of Yiddish actors he saw in the 1910s, is fed by his criticism of what the writer does, feeding on the marrow of his race, doing 'research' as his sleuth-hound puts it. He turns suspicion on himself. Brecht might have scorned the exactly dreamed precision of Kafka's stories, but he also noted that Kafka had all the attributes of a great teacher: without a society to inspire, his apparently ingrained Confucianism ended up as 'mere' literature. Kafka noted this about himself too, as a postcard in 1916 to his fiancée Felice praising the landscape around the spa town of Marienbad attests: 'I think that if I were Chinese and were going home (in fact I am Chinese and am going home), I would soon have to find a way to come back here.' The myth of the Way (the Chinese *tao*) was of overriding importance to Kafka, though once again he put a stumbling block in his way. There may be a goal, he told his notebook, but there is no way of reaching it.

Everything is weighed in terms of what we might call its social utility value, and writing is found wanting. Doctoring, too. The Enlightenment philosopher Diderot speculates, in one of his dialogues, about the secret kinship between criminals and artists (though it has always been easier, as the career of the Marquis de Sade illustrates, to commit atrocities in the head than write good novels); the villagers sketched out in *A Country Doctor* also seem to regard the doctor, despite his apparent bond to the life of the community, as a kind of miscreant: he rides across the social order, he flaunts his individuality in the face of common values, his opinions are dissentient. He is a kind of antinomian. Society punishes the doctor for the gratification he derives from his odd hours of service by making him an outlaw. Butcher, executioner, barber and surgeon used all to be trades which, dealing with blood and guts, carried a weight of social opprobrium. As dignified as he is ponderous, Kafka's country doctor mimes solidarity with tradition even while knowing his acts follow—and sometimes even parade—the logic of enlightenment. His sense of impending persecution has the touchy tone heard so often in the confessions and letters of Rousseau, assertive even while it looks defensively over its shoulder: the citizen of Geneva may have contributed to the *Encyclopédie*, but he was also one of literature's most thankless characters, and father to the very Kafkaesque conviction that the forms and conventions of civilised life occasion our ills.

In relation to the criminal or miscreant, the doctor's moral vanity makes him even more of a target. He is, we realise with a start, brother to the man on the rack in Kafka's terrible dramatisation of the condemned prisoner who learns his sentence on his person, *The Penal Colony,* a story we know to have been inspired in part by his reading of the infamous case of the French army officer Alfred Dreyfus, found guilty of a trumped-up charge of treason in 1894, and banished to the prison colony of Devil's Island. In his story Kafka's chosen instrument of torture appears to be a Gutenberg screw press.

It is hardly incidental, then, that the first bodies authorised by the Church for dissection in Renaissance anatomy theatres were those of the condemned, still warm from the gallows. Ontologically, and certainly in the mystical body of the Church, they would always be men, no matter how violently extirpated from the social body. Nonetheless, the logic of the grudging consent from the pulpit amounts to an imprecation: cut up your own then, Men of Science! Let your knowledge bleed!

Hidden in full view

Lastly, it strikes me that the patient on the bed bears his wound like Jacob who, after wrestling the night through with the angel on the mountain, calls on the angel to bless him—even if it might seem like a curse to Kafka. There seems to be a buried reference to the Biblical scene in his first 'real' piece of writing, 'The Judgement' (1912), in which the seemingly invalid father hooks up his shirt, aping his son's fiancée, and displays his 'war wound'. His act of indecent exposure seems calculated to call into question his son's very manhood. Kafka mentions a similarly suggestive episode in his travel diaries. Planning to visit Paris in October 1910, he was forced to shelve his plans and stay in Prague due to a severe attack of furunculosis (boils on his backside) and writes, 'a brief fainting spell deprived me of the pleasure of bawling the doctor out. I had to lie down on the sofa, and during that time—it was very odd—I felt so much like a girl that I tried with my fingers to tug down my skirt.'

The 'wound', in fact, was Kafka's word for the experience of writing: his first story forced him to recognise his nature as a writer. He was one of those self-doubters, like his great predecessor, the Danish theologian Søren Kierkegaard, who kept open 'the wound of the negative' so that trust might close it again in some kind of natural healing process. Kafka's, however, was a mortal wound, since, as he wrote to Max Brod, a writer 'dies (or doesn't really live) and is perpetually sorry for himself'.

Most disconcertingly of all, for those of us who take pleasure in reading Kafka, in trusting him as a writer, is the extraliterary dimension his writing has acquired. Kafka is now a prophet. J.P. Stern, late Professor of German at University College London, has pointed out that there is a resemblance between Kafka's description of the wound and the unappetising use of natural metaphors in anti-Semitic propaganda, the most notorious being a passage in Hitler's *Mein Kampf* about scandals in Vienna before the First World War in which he talks about 'the leech on the Nation's body'. The German word for insect or vermin (Ungeziefer) which

Kafka uses to describe Gregor Samsa in *Metamorphosis* is one of the terms the Nazis later used to stigmatise the Jews.

What is interpreted as Kafka's clairvoyance is surely his ability to grasp the stock phrases and figures of speech conventionally reserved for conveying mental and emotional states with the mental equivalent of the country doctor's forceps: not as metaphor, but as words of literal intent, however much they try to hide—like the hapless patient's wound—in full view. That is what prophets do: they read the impersonal logic that stands behind the most commonplace utterances. And they have to be right if they're not to be wrong.

Kafka shows us, sometimes in amazing detail, the intellectual contortions and special inner pleading that afflict people who try to make sense of the arbitrary. What is most striking perhaps about his victims is that they rarely take any steps to avoid the fate they seem to have expected from the first. The unthinkable is a category of monster: it is what we never care to think about.

A prosthetic life

These days the country doctor's model patient can be found in any old family: he's probably looking forward to being able to walk again in a few weeks now his hip is a vanadium and titanium sphere bonded to his femoral shaft, for a good fifteen years at least, with biocompatible epoxy resin. Writing to Brod from the sanatorium in the Erzgebirge just after he had completed *A Country Doctor* in 1917, Kafka dwells at length on his uncle's imperturbable cheeriness and aptitude for life in the country, and suggests that this kind of life might have tempted him too—'the way a slight rustling madness can make a person contented, thinking it the melody of life'. But at thirty-four, with questionable lungs and even more questionable relationships, he decides he has no right to such an expectation. And besides, flight from the paternal line is in that desire; the compelling nocturnal spectacle of Hope grappling with his Father.

Perhaps only the anorexic Kafka could have dignified his beefy middle-aged dad in such a way, as if he were calling the toss with the Wrestler of Genesis, 'who touched the hollow of Jacob's thigh in the sinew of the hip'.

The wound had done its work. It was a moribund man who rehearsed a normal life with Dora in the last few weeks of the only life he had. 'Franz is cheery and in good shape', appends Dora to one of Franz's last letters; and a simple country doctor might wonder at the affection with which he addresses his parents, especially the father he made stand in so often as tormentor; at how he comes to accept his body and his manhood, even as his illness, and not its metaphor, kills him.

As for his uncle, we have a story that sees through him: the photograph reproduced in the Wagenbach book has him sitting on a metal skeleton with the power of about twenty thoroughbreds, thighs urging it forward, knuckles clenched on the throttle, while four female helpers, including Kafka's favourite sister Ottla—the one who encouraged Franz so much to quit the parental house in Prague, and sustained him with regular food-packets in his last months with Dora in Berlin—smile triumphantly through the long exposure time in front of what may well have been Uncle Siegfried's camera too.

In the photo Uncle Siegfried's NSU Cantilever is actually resting on its rear stand—poised for a moment in time, like the four human figures in the picture, on its own two legs.

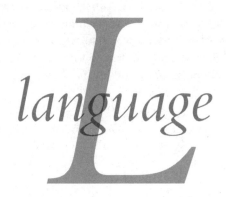

language

Is there Life on Earth?

SOME OBSERVATIONS ON TECHNICAL LANGUAGE

*Technology is on course to achieve such a degree
of perfection that humans will get by without themselves.*
— Stanisław Jerzy Lec

For an information technologist what you and I engage in on a daily, more or less unselfconscious basis is 'fuzzy discourse'. What is fuzzy discourse?—try talking to someone with a microphone nearby or read something you've dictated in a hurry and you'll see in an instant what's fuzzy about it: lots of throat-clearing enunciations, phatic slab-words, trailing conjunctions, broken-backed metaphors. Linguists call these 'discourse markers'. Language doesn't flow; it comes in stops and starts. Sometimes it looks like the angel wrestled by Jacob, and smashed to bits on hard ground. This idea was once expressed supremely well by Karl Kraus, the one-man Viennese cabarettist and publisher who never tired of telling German-speakers how naked the emperor was: 'in no language is it so difficult to make oneself understood as in language'.

For information technologists aiming to corner the market in voice recognition systems and who probably wouldn't give a hoot for Karl Kraus, what happens in daily life must be horrifying.

Like us, information technologists more or less speak a language. Inside the doors of their specialism, they cultivate what is properly called an ideolect, and they're presumably realistic enough to know that a galactic interlanguage in which everyone can talk shop and be understood is about as pertinent a prospect as finding an Elsevier dictionary in the next world. What is language using us for if not to sow misunderstanding, humankind's rogue creative principle? In the tongues of angels, however, who never squabble (even if they disobey God), words exactly embrace their objects. Since we can't pretend to speak High Angelic, what we have in our world is a vehicular subvariety of English called Tech Talk. TT—acronym is as much a quick fix in TT as elsewhere, witness Chomsky's LAD or 'language acquisition device'—is a way of giving structure and functional rigour to the fuzziness of everyday life. Language finds a way of saying what it needs to; that is an axiom which introduces us to quite a different set of assumptions from those of the famous Sapir-Whorf hypothesis, suggesting that we can't think what our languages can't say (Orwell's Newspeak).

TT is a variety of discourse based on algorithms, an algorithm being an arborescent decision evaluation process template (ADEPT), a very distant and parodic offshoot of the Tree of Knowledge. Doctors, for example, use algorithms all the time (and they're published in family-tree format in doctors' journals and in the backpages of books called *Five Minutes for the Patient* to make it easier for them to be slid under the little plastic protectors doctors keep on their desks) as a way of not having to think too hard (or even to think at all). You turn up with symptom A: question: do you have contextually associated symptom B: question: Is it provoked by C; and so on, until diagnosis emerges by a process of exclusion. Or perhaps exhaustion. This method derives from Sydenham in the seventeenth-century. In his attempt to identify clinical phenomena as closely as possible in the hope of establishing common signs and symptoms, he adopted the method used by the natural historian to describe species. But reading through the hiererachy of almost legalistic specifications in the Diagnostic and Statistical Manual (DSM) of Mental Disorders, Fourth Edition (*the*

American manual of psychiatric disorders) can leave an innocently inexplicit rule-deductionist quite dizzy at the multiplication of species (no threat of extinction here); and WHO's *Manual of the International Statistical Classification of Diseases, Injuries, and Causes of Death* contrives to be appalling and fascinating in equal parts. The philosopher Lichtenberg could no longer claim, as he did in his scrapbook for 1789, that 'anxieties and gloomy thoughts [are not] among the register of diseases: this is very wrong'. Every distress has its technical idiom. This is section E 980–989, 'Injury undetermined whether accidentally or purposely inflicted':

E 980   Poisoning by solid or liquid substances, undetermined whether accidentally or purposely inflicted

E981   Poisoning by gases in domestic use, undetermined whether accidentally or purposely inflicted

E982   Poisoning by other gases, undetermined whether accidentally or purposely inflicted

E983   Hanging, strangulation or suffocation, undetermined whether accidentally or purposely inflicted

E984   Submersion [drowning], undetermined whether accidentally or purposely inflicted

E985   Injury by firearms and explosives, undetermined whether accidentally or purposely inflicted

E986   Injury by cutting and piercing, undetermined whether accidentally or purposely inflicted

E987   Falling from high place, undetermined whether accidentally or purposely inflicted

E988   Injury by other and unspecified means, undetermined whether accidentally or purposely inflicted

E989   Late effects of injury, undetermined whether accidentally or purposely inflicted

I like that Biblical 'falling from high place'. You might make a mess on the ground, citizen, but there won't be any ink stains on the death certificate.

Who uses Tech Talk? We all do, in fact, although some professional groups are more likely to use it on a systematic basis than
others. Its pedigree goes back further, and into stranger recesses,
than you might suppose. The Church and its doctrinalists were
a founding source. Shakespeare, in a proto-Tech Talk scene
from the Scottish play, has Macbeth translate himself down for
the intellectually challenged in the front rows of the Globe with
his hand that 'will rather / The multitudinous seas incarnadine,
/ Making the green one red'; and Dr Johnson fingers another
culprit: Sir Thomas Browne, coiner of such otiose titles as *Pseu-
dodoxia Epidemica*, whom he chastens for pouring in 'a multitude
of exotick words'. Or Dr Johnson himself, clearly not having
heard the joke about lots of little holes joined up with string: 'any
thing reticulated or decussated, at equal distances, with interstices
between the intersections' (a net).

The first book in English to be called a dictionary, by Henry
Cockeram in 1623, was in fact subtitled *an Interpreter of Hard
English Words*; although the first 'conceptual dictionary', in which
words are arranged in groups by their meaning, was first promulgated by Bishop John Wilkins in his *Essay towards a Real Character
and a Philosophical Language* (1668). Wilkins wanted to give a more
meaningful, structuring sense to functional variety, to represent
the multiplicity of relationships, both potential and actual. The
nineteenth century—the century of the OED—was the formative age of TT, possibly because people still knew their classics.
Think of Bouvard and Pécuchet, and the sixteen hundred books
Flaubert had to read before his two *bonshommes* knew they had to
give up trying to understand the world. If we look under Balzac's
valiant attempts to classify society much like a zoologist we find,
not surprisingly, Linnaeus and Buffon, but also Goethe, with his
unrealised 'novel about the universe'. In his *Manifesto*, Zola—who
thought Balzacian classification outdated in relation to his more
modern notion of the novelist as experimentalist—actually quotes
pages and pages of Claude Bernard, the physiologist. And surely
Joyce's overweening ambition to capture a day in all its nuances—a
day as a book, with nothing omitted—is a TT ambition? 'The
infinite lattiginous scintillating uncondensed milky way' turns up
somewhere or other in *Ulysses*. More recently James Fenton, a
poet with a very large forebrain, bravely went on record about

his wish to provide poetry with a language for the future: this he evidenced once in a very Victorian series of 'found' poems called *Exempla*, one of which replicates the weird beauty of the following line from *Mycologia* (Vol. 60): 'I deal in minutiae, / Not with the fungus growing on the low walls but its / Globose vesiculate hyaline conidia'. Taxonomies, as Fenton suggests, are not entirely the arid, abstract exercises some people might write them off as being; they are densely clustered verbal theories about what they represent. The outstanding natural history book *Five Kingdoms: An Illustrated Guide to the Phyla of Life on Earth*, by Margulis and Schwartz, is just such an exemplum. Or, as the Collins' guide *Birds of Britain and Europe* explains:

> Scientists classify all animals in a series of groupings, starting with 22 phyla and proceeding downwards through classes, orders, families (ending in *-idae*), subfamilies (ending in *-inae*) and genera to the actual species, below which there are sometimes subspecies or races based on geographical variation. Birds belong to the phylum Cordata, along with the mammals, reptiles and fishes, and are themselves distinguished as the class Aves. With the Aves class, there are 27 orders of living birds, much the largest of which is the Passeriformes, loosely known as song birds, perching birds, or Passerines. The passerines comprise more than half the known bird species of the world, and more than a third of the 154 bird families. They are all terrestrial and very diverse in shape and form, but generally adapted to perching in trees and often have a very well developed song.

It was the achievement of a poet—the Russian poet Osip Mandelstam, who actually resembled a passerine according to his wife in her memoir about their difficult life in the Soviet Union—to find a formula for the figure standing in the shadows behind them all, dangerous Mr Darwin, 'who possessed the courage to be prosaic precisely because he had so much to say and did not feel obliged to express rapture or gratitude to anyone'.

That list is, of course, a very selective, partial identification of only those names visible from my writing desk. It overlooks most of the real actors and movers, a list which should probably include the Vietnam War, aerospace scientists, Buckminster Fuller, and the impersonal militaristic restructuring of consciousness required for the smooth running of batch processing, QA/QC, and alphanumeric systems. (The fêted non-gametic 'photocopy' sheep Dolly is much more a product of commercial interests than of disinterested scientific curiosity, and as such should properly be called Dolly™. I hardly have to force the invidious parallel.)

At a deeper level, English's schizoid nature is a tireless generator of task-specific nomenclature, its primary input source being, of course, the Norman Conquest. There's a whiff of clergyman and cleric in TT, aureate classicisms being intoned in a draughty place above the din of Germanic monosyllables. This forking of the tongue is all the more obvious in historically more innocent forms of English: the effect of all those German immigrants settling in the mid-west on American English usage has been far-reaching. Germans are as likely to say 'Personenkraftwagen' (PKW in its quick fix form) as 'Auto'. Even a simple bricks-and-mortar conjunction like '*oder*' (or) is often supplanted with the toothy 'beziehungweise', which carries a more apparent charge of order and rank, although in written language it bristles as 'bzw.'. Technical people have always marvelled at those ultra-concise German compound terms like 'Wärmeleitfähigkeitsdetektor', which is a device for measuring heat conductivity, or the nippy 'Kontrastmittellösung' used by radiologists to designate a radio-opaque solution for enhancing X-rays. In old Fiji, before the missionaries, rugged warriors used to eat the brains of their defeated enemies in order to absorb their *mana*; those who won the last war did the same, but being too sophisticated to eat flesh, cannibalised mere mouthfuls of air. Twentieth-century Americans are no slouchers when it comes to Chicago Dutch. Webster's dictionary insists on plain speaking, but put American English in a bureaucratic high-tech environment and listen to the way it goes into phase transition. Gadgeteer Optimism, forsooth.

Less is more. If TT has one governing principle, it is this: communicate with parsimony, do not indulge in circumlocution. Be rigorous, the world is object-rich. Primo Levi once pointed out how many chemical compounds there are—over two million— and if chemistry, as compared to alchemy, has been able to build its house on phlogisticon and antinomy and mercury, predicting the existence of elements from their hypothetical place in the

Periodic Table long before they had been identified, it is because each compound is part of a vast interlocking structure in which one thing conditions and is conditioned by its neighbours. Named insect species reach roughly the same total. No parole for this *langue*.

Texpressions are often misused in their guise as a sublanguage of impersonal agency, most prominently and perniciously by four-star American generals to baffle the immediate enemy called the press corps. Human Remains Pouch or the squeaky-sounding Smart Weapon are euphemisms of abysmal cuteness; the helicopter machine guns that mowed down Vietnamese peasants in the war were called Puff the Magic Dragon. Euphemism and death always go together: the Greek Furies, older even than Zeus, were always referred to in conversation as the Eumenides, the Kindly Ones, just as Hades was Pluto, Mr Rich. Alfred Nobel, founder of the prize that bears his name and another man who wasn't short of a bob, was a distinguished euphemist: he called the nitrate compound discovered in his own laboratory in 1866 'safety powder', the rest of the world preferring to call it dynamite. Tech Talk, it may be noted, offers little resistance to being driven to that kind of extreme, exploding people in the same way a draughtsman explodes a technical drawing. In Dante's *Inferno*, all the damned distort language to their own ends, and the worst can only babble. Consider, in passing, the strangeness of the world(s) we live in when one side in the Gulf War issued flowery old-style parafundities like 'Mother of All Battles' while the other constipated us with the verbal equivalent of fast food.

Like all mythic languages then, TT has two faces. It shouldn't adulterate or be adulterated by after-dinner orotundities or political doublespeak, though it will be. It is capable of being both radical novelty *and* ancient repressive instrument for upholding the firm. Perhaps I can hazard a definition or two: it is a technocratic task-specific semiotic paradigm transfer system, with the useful spin-off effect of ensuring primary user status enhancement. Well, that's just obscurantist jargon, you're saying. Not entirely. Jargon is a prophylactic *against* understanding, a meta-language semantically too broad for what it's describing (go and listen to any university sociologist obfuscating if you want to know what physics envy is); an honest TT word-stacker is desperate for you to hear the whisper, clank, glug and scrape of things. He wants you to show you his collection of fast fluid-attenuated inversion recovery (FLAIR) and half-Fourier acquisition single-shot turbo spin-echo (HASTE) images of your head in the MRI sequencer. He wants, in short, to say something non-fuzzy about the things which give TT its oomph. (Whether he wants, or even needs you to understand what he does at work is another matter.) Language is stripped back to the denotative. It's a question of economics in a situation in which the advantages of the kind of mental hygiene that TT confers are never under question. Good TT enlarges the bounds of comprehension even as it yields up the true intricacy of things. Indeed, TT is anti-entropic. Why call a spade a spade when it's a spatulate pedally-applied dirt extractor?

Latin and Greek provide the core terms with which to start the algorithmic compounding. 'Organism' is an old favourite (though Richard Dawkins, biologist-cum-fundamentalist of the selfish gene, isn't happy using that—as it were—tried and tested Texpression: he opts instead for the more patently declarative 'vehicle'). 'Matrix' is a more recent buzzword. These are the important root-terms, the substantive building-blocks. Word lego, if you like. They're also usually the easiest to define. Take the following examples: 'icon', 'cell', 'node', 'paradigm', 'habitat', 'system', 'entity', 'complex'. What they define is the nature of the system; general and non-specific, they often lack the true cutting edge of TT. Other more specific core terms can be used but depend on the degree of professional specificity required: 'fractionator', 'donor', 'buffer', 'assay', for instance, the first two being active core terms, the latter two passive. Cystic fibrosis, for example, is due to a mutation of the cystic fibrosis transmembrane conductance regulator gene on chromosome 7, as it happens a mutation 1 in 20 of us carry as heterozygotes. 'Steady-state', the term in pharmacokinetics (not cosmology) that designates the period during which continued intake maintains a constant effective drug level in the plasma while wobbling over the dash like a drunk man trying to regain his balance, is a personal favourite.

The busy terms are the common specific epithets (CSE) and modifiers. These form an agglutinate around the core terms, and the descriptive power of the Tech Talk locution is directly dependent on what is stacked in front of the substantive. Some are structural, some qualifying, some processive. One of the great advantages of Tech Talk (and English generally) is that nouns can be press-ganged to work as adjectives. They may be static or dynamic, depending on the object. They can be subdivided in the best French schoolbook fashion (*Penser/Classer*, the title Georges Perec gave to one of his books) into as many classifications as you can come up with: form, colour, state, origin, etc. Words like 'quasi-static', 'pleomorphic', 'homogeneous', 'randomised' are a few instances of the terms that separate the expert Tech Talkers from the greenhorns. William Gibson's latest cybernovel mentions a 'Rodel-van Erp primary biomolecular programming module C-slash-7A'. Ben Marcus' disinformatively meaningful first book *The Age of Wire and String* devotes itself entirely to recalibrating language, creating a world in which the seasons, for instance, are defined *legally*, and words, intoned or revoked from the atmosphere, permanently alter its temperature. This is how he defines his title:

> AGE OF WIRE AND STRING, THE: Period in which English science devised abstract parlance system based on the flutter pattern of string and wire structures placed over the mouth during speech. Patriarch systems and figures, including Michael Marcuses, were also constructed in this period—they are the only fathers to outlast their era.

Here the classics come into their own. Take medicine (again). A good Tech Talk word used by doctors to describe the condition of neurotic patients who present with symptoms for which there is no objective cause is somatisation (also called Briquet's syndrome, an eponym being almost as quick a fix as an acronym). Linguistically, doctors somaticise all the time. Who can resist the semiotically enriched resonance of CSE like 'visceral', 'glossal', 'talar', 'diaphoretic', 'desquamating' and 'verruciform' once, like the medieval doctor, he has licked them with his tongue? Only Californian patients, in my experience, have ever been known to drop these words into a casual conversation with their physicians, though as a Limousin student explained to the startled Pantagruel

in Rabelais' great novel, 'my genius is not aptly nate, as this flati-
gious nebulon asserts, to excoriate the cuticle of our vernacular
Gallic, but vice-versally I gnave opere, and by sail and oar I enite
to locuplete it from the latinicome redundance' (Book 2, Chapter
6, Cohen's translation). It is only when Gargantua grabs him by
the throat that he stops trying to 'talk Parisian'.

Since the agglutinating can become very starchy, it's quite
common to add a few colourful but TT-specific qualifiers at the
start of the locution. 'Binary' is excellent TT, though 'on-off'
is acceptable too, as a concession to Anglo-Saxon monosyl-
labic directness. In fact, as whimsically Anglo-Saxon as you like,
provided the ordinary connotation of the qualifier only has a weak
force—'keyhole limpet haemocyanin' (KLH), 'zigzag DNA' and
other immunological and genetic engineering terms provide
good examples of how vernacular is conscripted to make function obvious through description. Some of the signal terms are
the smallest. 'Pre-' and 'post-' can be found everywhere. Other
prefixes go out in pairs like the animals from the Ark: 'dys-/eu-',
'macro-/micro-', 'inter-/intra-', 'ante-/retro-', so on and so forth.

Try it yourself (Edward Tenner's pioneering chapbook *Tech-
Speak* is an amusing guide for those who wish to learn how to coin
their own non-stochastic Texpressions using what he quaintly calls
his 'crystal seeding rules'). Everyone else is doing it, even if it has to
be pointed out to him. Look around your house and you'll probably find a few consumer-devotional TT icons. My wife's face
lotion advertises itself as a 'high intensity moisture gel for thirsty
skin'. It's easy to be blinded by science on Planet Skincare, where
the price of what is essentially a mixture of oils and water is directly
proportional to the number of Texpressions on the package. You
will almost certainly have used a 'serial interface' or a 'multiuser
docking port' on a computer. Everyone knows what a cathode ray
tube is. The raw materials for a leap into TT hyperprecision are all
around us. Open the fridge and take out a carton of milk. Now
say it in TT: a fixed-form bovine lacteal recipient. And probably
UHT at that. As Barthes noted in one of his exquisite mythologies,
the world of advertisement offers 'a whole Molièresque vocabulary, updated perhaps by a touch of scientism'. Not least for fast
moving consumer goods (FMCG), where language seems to shift
almost as fast as the goods.

What effect does TT have in a real-time anthropoid interface profession like medicine—is it mystifying and inhumane? That's a chicken-and-egg question that goes back to the Whorf-Sapir hypothesis, in the light of which a paper-pusher's locution like 'negative patient care outcome' represents metaphysical degree zero. Personally I don't use much TT in medicine since patients would rightly regard it as a kind of periphrastic high talk, heaping of insult on injury, or just noises off; though when I work as a TT translator in the quiet bits between patients or deep into the night, I have no option. I simply observe the familiar suddenly become exceedingly strange, professional vices become oddly militant. I find it interesting though that the compiler of the most famous 'conceptual dictionary' of all, Peter Marc Roget's *Thesaurus* (1852), was a Manchester doctor; here is Roget's (or rather the 5th edition's updated) entry 887.6 under the generic heading UNIMPORTANCE:

> **an insignificancy**, an inessential, a marginal matter *or* affair, a trivial *or* paltry affair, a small *or* trifling *or* minor matter, **no great matter**; a little thing, *peu de chose* <Fr>, hardly *or* scarcely anything, matter of no importance *or* consequence, matter of indifference; **a nothing**, a big nothing, a naught, a mere nothing, nothing in particular, nothing to signify, nothing to speak *or* worth speaking of, nothing to think twice about, nothing to boast of, nothing to write home about, thing of naught, *rien du tout* <Fr>, nullity, nihility; **technicality**, mere technicality

Compare such an entry, to take one at random, with the main causes of dementia in adults:

> Alzheimer's disease; hypothyroidism, subacute combined degeneration of the cord; pellagra; hypoparathyroidism; multiple cerebral infarction; alcohol/Wenicke-Korsakoff syndrome; intracranial mass, hydrocephalus (including subdural haematoma); chronic traumatic encephalopathy; Huntington's disease; multiple sclerosis; spongiform encephalopathy; progressive supranuclear palsy; general paralysis of the insane; drug or heavy metal poisoning; post-anoxia or -hypoglycaemia; chronic

hepatic encephalopathy; AIDS encephalopathy; uraemia, rare metabolic disorders, e.g. Wilson's disease.

Notice too how easily the technical imagination—not an oxymoron, as this essay has tried to prove—obliterates itself. I would prefer to leave the moralising about language to Orwellians and other prescriptivists for whom the technotalkative, as Nicholson Baker has called it, is sheer torture. TT always wraps itself in a nimbus of plausibility. It aims for precision, control and efficiency, and it shouldn't be surprising if that naively upbeat Enlightenment impulse to reveal the material nature of the world becomes more and more ramified as it broadens. That is its peculiar illusion: all language is equidistant from reality. Only the words are different. Language speaks, and we have to be scrupulous in attending to it. That is essentially a religious attitude; it comes down to us from the pre-Socratics whose *logos*, the ordering principle of the universe, was not some reality supposed to lie behind words, but the thing itself. It is surely some kind of phylogenetic guarantee that language can never be quite as supine as we fear it might be, even if Karl Kraus was known to deplore the fact that half a man could write a whole sentence. He also said: 'The closer you look at a word, the further it looks back at you from.'

Are platitudes all we have? Has a transcendent technology found us helpless, stricken without our clichés? That proud American word 'know-how' long ago—to my ear at least—started to acquire an ironic British feel. The materials of life have changed, language trails behind, and the old general-purpose terms get stretched and bent to the new circumstances. It's a kind of cognitive dissonance we're all fluent with, since we accept it as a trade-off: the price of advancing knowledge is that we, too, become objects of that knowledge. There's nothing inherently scientific about TT's lego principle of reality, any more than biology is a field of study that looks at 'life'. Chuck Jones, the American cartoonist who brought the trickster sagas into the age of Looney Tunes, had Marvin the Martian trying to vaporize our planet with his 'Iludium pew-36 Explosive Space Modulator'. The McDonald's operators' manual, nanotechnology and ISO 9002 certificates must have been the reinforcements.

Finding a language for life on Earth probably has a lot to

do with a history of rising expectations, AT/GC ratios on the human genome and those shadowy double-agents called translators who spend a lot of time transforming apparently value-free words from one stunned language into another. It's the Steptoe & Son approach to things: cobbling them together and making them up while gleaming new technologies become as capriciously disdainful of mere mortals as Zeus was in his heyday. My latest reading of the pandemonium model tells me that computer logic now incorporates, of all things, non-linear logic: instead of a strict $A+B=C$ approach, the silicon matrices are programmed to admit that $A+B\approx C$. What that fuzzy little sign means, I suppose, is that facts settle at their own cognitive level too, one that exposes how much we're enmeshed in them, while those other facts of our world called machines, once self-evident antonyms to anything human, now seem so unaccountably lively.

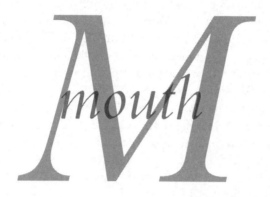

Tell Me about Teeth

A DOCTOR LOOKS AT A DENTIST

It was Elias Canetti who threw down the challenge: 'To write about teeth. Just try!'

Canetti's epigraph is the opener for an article on teeth by the American essayist Eliot Weinberger, one of the writings in his exquisite book *Karmic Traces*. In an enjoyably bizarre reflection on the problems of non-occlusion in his pet rabbit, he notices, as I have too, that while many writers seem to earn their keep by being qualified doctors, he couldn't think of a single writer who puts in hours as a dentist. Teeth, Weinberger reasons, are too often identified with power, or the lack of it: 'the sickness of the tooth and its subsequent extraction have tended to be viewed allegorically rather than as revelatory of human nature'.

In fact, dentists perch too close to the cutting edge of sarcasm to entertain immodest thoughts about having been specially endowed—as physicians so often like to boast—with extrahuman humane concerns. How can you believe the soul is a butterfly when the human breath is so foetid? Dentists ought to make good satirists, even if they all too often end up as the butt of satire. The Russian poet Osip Mandelstam, who was banished to the Gulag after daring to write a satirical poem about Stalin, had a thing about the buzzing of the dental burr (his teeth weren't in such good shape either) and wrote sarcastically about loving 'dentists for their artistry, their wide horizons and their tolerance of ideas' (*The Egyptian Stamp*).

Perhaps the bigger problem with being a dentist is that you can't have a conversation with your patients, at least not much of a verbal exchange. Anything a patient says with a drainage pipe, cotton wool and gloved fingers in mouth is going to sound strangulated. It's no way to learn about the roots of social problems.

It seems appropriate enough that Canetti, who spent twenty years of his life in London writing his unclassifiable book *Crowds and Power*, should seize on a symbol which, if you watch a lot of television, seems to be what television is best at revealing. In the world of show-biz TV, people smile, and they smile because they know that figuratively at least they're having you for breakfast; and the more the showmaster flashes his credentials (and everybody knows it's a faked smile) the more pitiless it all seems. This stopper-rod assembly, this fender-bar, this enamel xylophone of incisors, canines and premolars that makes a mouth: after years of orthodontic corralling and straightening, it may be perfect to the millimetre, every tooth a regular tombstone—but which tombstone ever had this effulgence, this phosphorescent veneer, this *whiteness*?

There are mouths that fill screens. Some of them are macrognathic too, gleaming Chrysler fenders, enormous lower jaws that can barely contain all the teeth. As the French sociologist Jean Baudrillard once remarked, 'Americans may have no identity, but they do have wonderful teeth.' The whiteness of American teeth is virtue itself; and the Italian writer Curzio Malaparte, in one of his novels about the end of the Second World War, was haunted by the dental arcade 'that every American, as he steps smiling into his grave, projects like a final salute to the world of the living'. It was of course an American marketeer, Claude C. Hopkins, who got people to brush their teeth regularly with Pepsodent in the early years of the twentieth century (and allegedly inspired Willem de Kooning's famous series *Woman*, in which each just-about-recognisable female form sports formidable teeth). Now Americans spend three billion dollars every year on aesthetic dentistry alone.

It had all been prefigured by Edgar Allan Poe, who wrote an especially creepy story, 'Berenice', about a man obsessed with a beautiful consumptive girl who, like a ghoulish version of the Cheshire cat, shrinks back to her teeth: his nightmare was illustrated by Odilon Redon in a charcoal drawing of 1883, which shows two rows of gleaming teeth suspended in front of a shelf of books to which they impart the most spectral light.

Franz Kafka, in one of his meditations on power and powerlessness, sees teeth where nobody else does. 'It was an ordinary day; it bared its teeth at me; I too was held by the teeth and couldn't squirm out of their grip; I didn't know how they were holding me, for they weren't clenched; nor did I see them in the form of the two rows of a dental arcade, but merely some teeth here and some there. I wanted to hold on to them and vault over them, but I didn't succeed in doing so.'

The steeplechase through the graveyard might not have worked out for Kafka, but periodontal medicine has come on leaps and bounds since his time. Nobody has to lose all their teeth at the age of eighteen these days, as half the inhabitants of Glasgow did in 1900 (many still lose their teeth even now, though perhaps not all at once). The journalist Ian Jack, who comes from the other side of Scotland, wrote an off-putting piece for the *Guardian* newspaper about his father arranging to have all his teeth removed before he was fifty, and spitting them out one by one into a bucket, while the dentist stood by; his mother had long since been edentulous. Being a practical man, his father thought it would make life easier not having any more teeth to worry about.

The German mystic Jakob Boehme would have sympathised with Jack's father's decision: in his writings he suggested that the prelapsarian Adam needed no teeth for eating the 'Paradisicall fruit'. It is quite a thought: Adam and Eve were masticating with their gums until the Fall. (Of course, they hardly needed to consume either, having nothing as revolting as entrails.) But the deep metaphysical problem with teeth comes from a different direction: you need them not just to eat but to speak.

The Jack family's loss of dentition was nothing unusual in Scotland. In the early twentieth century conservative dentistry was almost unheard of except in Scandinavia and the United States. Prostheses ('falsers' or 'wally-dugs' in Glasgow), bridges and implants successively replaced teeth rotted by time's subtle sugars. Some scientists even began to think of caries as a slow-acting infectious disease. But who's thinking caries? Now whitening techniques ('customize your bright, white smile') help to give the impression that we are a generation not just of perfect teeth, but perfect *tout court*. The Smile Design Center in Los Angeles makes a livelihood from exploiting the fact that the impeccable smile is a social marker, and not just in Hollywood. No need to suffer the stain of tobacco: fingers might be yellow, but teeth can be brushed and polished clean, and even veneered. All of the members of the immigrant families in Zadie Smith's *White Teeth* have what the novel's title advertises. They are poised, as it were, between the strong natural teeth of people who have yet to meet the refinements of civilisation and civilisation's ability to provide extraordinarily refined dental aftercare.

Stomatology would seem to be a brazen business then. Yet, strangely enough, the suspicion remains that these perfect teeth are hiding something. Perhaps they're not really *morally* perfect teeth? They smile at you but mean to tear you limb from limb. '*Und der Haifisch, der hat Zähne, und die trägt er im Gesicht*', wrote Bertolt Brecht in his famous song about Mack the Knife. The shark has teeth, and he sports them in his face—sure, and they don't always stay in the oral cavity. Giorgio Pressburger writes in his story 'Teeth' that his obsession with teeth began the day when, as a child of six, he saw an old actor begging in the street who, at the end of his routine, whipped out his false teeth in order to bag the sympathy coin. I can only imagine that his sense of pity was sharpened by a streak of that other moral sentiment, disgust. In one of his novels Philip Roth is pleased to inform us that the mouth in its very origins is also a hiding place, being derived from the same germinal tissue in the embryo as the genitals.

Humans are nothing if not dialectical. How else could baring the teeth, the most unambiguously aggressive and hostile of facial expressions, qualify with the help of a few other changes in facial posture as the universal signal of friendliness and cooperation?

Darwin notices, in his remarkable other book *The Expression of the Emotions in Man and Animals* (1872), one of the first scientific books to be published with photographic illustrations, that the teeth are generally exposed by the raising of the upper lip under the action of the zygomatic major muscle. It was the pioneering French neurologist Duchenne who noticed that the genuine smile of enjoyment rather than just the frozen gesture of appeasement involved the action of the eye muscles in synchrony with the lip muscles. To grin, though, has two meanings: not only to smile, but also to draw back the lips in a grimace of leering displeasure or aggressive intent. In sneers of defiance, noted Darwin, the canine on one side only tends to be exposed (and it must be of interest to more than philosophers of the Cynical School that 'sneer' and 'snarl' are cognates, too).

When I eventually located that Canetti epigraph, on page 242 of his book of aphorisms *The Human Province*, I discovered what he had actually written was: 'To write *without* teeth. Just try!' Had that great 'Menschenfresser' (man-eater) Canetti left his falsers at home on one of his research raids on the old British Library? Was the haughtiest man in Hampstead down on his uppers? It was a Pressburger moment that cast Canetti's lifelong obsession with power relations in an entirely new light. Now it made sense to me why Canetti thought false teeth had something to do with dialectics. Dialectics are falsers which, if you use them to bite into a stone instead of a freshly baked loaf, will break, just as surely as the real ones.

If one of the events that define the end of history is that people no longer need to lose their teeth, it still needs to be said how many teeth have been lost in the course of history.

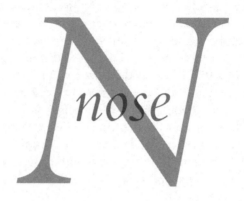

Hygiene of the Soul

SMELL AND THE MORAL SENTIMENTS

The nose is the supremely Shandean organ. Protruding, comic, hubristic, shiny, a zoological bizarrery, as plain as any fact can be yet somehow related to that other organ hidden in men's breeks (and the nostrils are allegedly in tantric relation to all sorts of hidden psychic zones in both sexes), it seems first to have butted in on polite society in the novel Dr Johnson so greatly disapproved of—'Nothing odd will do long', he growled of Laurence Sterne's *The Life and Opinions of Tristram Shandy, Gentleman*.

Johnson's antipathy to the nose carried over into his conversation: Boswell reports in chapter 39 of his biography *The Life of Dr Johnson* an unsuccessful attempt by a young controversialist to get the good Doctor to take on board the notion that the mind might body itself forth other than through the eye: 'A young gentleman present took up the argument against him, and maintained that no man ever thinks of the *nose of the mind*, not adverting that though that figurative sense seems strange to us, as very unusual, it is truly not more forced than Hamlet's "In my *mind's eye*, Horatio." He persisted much too long, and appeared to Johnson as putting himself forward as his antagonist with too much presumption; upon which he called to him in a loud tone, "What is it you are contending for, if you BE contending?"' At which belligerent retort the young man backs off, and the conversation switches, in spite of Boswell's support for the figurative novelty of the nose as the organ of sagacity, to a different subject. Johnson had conversationally tweaked the young man's nose, his punishment for having tried to be too 'nose-wise'.

But the young man was onto something. It was following their noses which, as recounted in Slawkenbergius' Tale in Book IV of *Tristram Shandy*, ended the independence of the people of Strasbourg, previously a free city under the Holy Roman German Empire until Louis XIV descended on Alsace with imperial ambitions in 1683. ''Twas not the *French*,—'twas CURIOSITY pushed open [the gates of the city]—The *French* indeed, who are ever upon the catch, when they saw the *Strasburgers*, men, women, and children, all marched out to follow the stranger's nose—each man followed his own, and marched in.' In an era when people were to be seen without noses at all (destroyed in the later stages of syphilis), noses are replaced as casually as if they were spectacles. Dr Slop, the extraordinary accoucheur, fashions one for Tristram from 'a piece of cotton and a thin piece of whalebone out of Susannah's stays'.

When it eventually got to St Petersburg in the early nineteenth century, the nose went rampant. Vladimir Nabokov called the trend 'olfactivism'. Gogol wrote a famous story called 'The Nose' (1834), in which a socially aware nose, sliced off by a barber, gains the autonomous life that normal noses sometimes think they are entitled to. Its former owner, the minor bureaucrat Kovalyov, spots it dressed up in a gold-braided uniform and, in the kind of ingratiating language befitting its status, requests an audience. This nose is having a successful career without Kovalyov, so it thumbs its nose at him. In another of his famous short-stories, 'The Diary of a Madman', we are told that noses have even managed to build a lunar civilisation. 'That's why we can't see our own noses: they are all on the moon.'

Perhaps Gogol wrote his story simply under the inspiration

of the Russian expression 'to get only nose' (*ostat'sia s nosom*). Its sense is not dissimilar to the English idiom that leaves you with only the shirt on your back: you've been taken in, reader, and lost face. Except that this face still has a nose on it.

At any rate, there is more than a hint in Gogol that the senses are becoming uncoupled, perhaps to their greater benefit. The German poet Rainer Maria Rilke, by way of contrast, was obsessed with exploring the 'gaps' between what he called the five fingers of the senses: in his poem 'Orpheus. Eurydice. Hermes' the god's sight runs ahead of him like a dog, but his hearing lags like a smell—the kind of smell that can linger the best part of a lifetime. When Odysseus returned from his twenty years' meander around the Aegean, the only member of his household to recognise him was his old dog Argos—Odysseus still stank of master.

The nose has a bottom. When we want to evoke the palpability of an experience (or, better said, its sheer immediacy prior to any perceptive analysis or stirrings of the will) it is to the nose we turn. Tolstoy, in *The Death of Ivan Ilyich*, likens talk about death, which polite society must overlook or ignore, to somebody blowing off in the drawing room.

Smell is the most reliable sentinel, the indisputable arbiter of the moral sentiments. It is the organ able to root out the genuine article. Johann Fischart, one of the earliest masters of modern German prose, wrote a poem in 1571 with the motto '*Sie haben Nasen und riechen's nit*' (You have noses and smell it not) to defend Luther against accusations that he and other Protestants supped with the Devil. The great Russian poet Osip Mandelstam put it like this, in his essay 'The Word and Culture': 'I sense an almost physically unclean goat-breath emanating from the enemies of the word. Here the argument which emerges last in any serious disagreement is fully appropriate: an adversary smells bad.' Smells flag up the corrupt, but smells are themselves potentially defiling. They can get beneath our guard and threaten total physical and moral debasement, and bring with them besides the unwelcome attentions of dogs and flies. Commander R. H. S. Bacon, who travelled in Benin, the site of one of the most disgraceful episodes in British colonial history and backdrop for Conrad's famous novella, *Heart of Darkness*, must have been holding his nose with one hand while holding his pen with the other: '...everywhere death, barbarity and blood, and smells that it hardly seems right for human beings to smell and yet live!'

That he could smell, even figuratively, the death-dealing on their hands lends an eerily reckless bravado to Isaac Babel's explanation to the same Mandelstam of his penchant for spending time in Moscow with the notoriously brutal members of the Cheka, Stalin's secret police. 'M. asked him if he wanted to touch the death they dealt in with his fingers. "No," he replied, "I don't want to touch it with my fingers—I just like to have a sniff and find out what it smells like."' Babel's curiosity, needless to say, brought him to a sticky end—he was shot by the same secret police after a summary trial in 1940. He became a victim of the new Soviet concept of death by quota.

So what kind of revelation is a smell?

In *Ecce Homo*, a whirlwind effort of three weeks' concentrated work in Turin even as he was losing his grip on his mind, Friedrich Nietzsche reviewed his life of philosophical vagabondage in some extraordinary rhapsodic and apocalyptic pages. In the final chapter of that final book, which bears the immodest but not inaccurate heading 'Why I am a Destiny', he writes: '*Revaluation of all values*: this is my formula for an act of supreme coming-to-oneself on the part of mankind which in me has become flesh and genius. It is my fate to have to be the first *decent* human being, to know myself in opposition to the mendaciousness of millennia... I was the first to *discover* the truth, in that I was the first to sense—*smell*—the lie as lie... My genius is in my nostrils... I contradict as has never been contradicted and am none the less the opposite of a negative spirit.'

There's a bitingly witty touch in that idea of himself as the first decent man, and an even subtler wit in the sarcastic notion of sniffing truth—doggish, excremental and ground-level in one guise, mercilessly refined use of an underused faculty in another. In his notebooks, Ludwig Wittgenstein, discussing the lack of pretension and humility of the Gospels as compared to the Pauline scriptures, flatly concludes his argument with the line, 'That is, so to speak, what my *nose* tells me.' Richard Hoggart wrote that

Orwell, who had to overcome an extremely fastidious (middle-class) sense of propriety in order to gather (lower-class) material for *The Road to Wigan Pier*, 'could *smell* his way through complex experiences'. Decades before him, Flaubert had been unable to sleep after having breathed the odour of the 'proletarians' in the omnibus (he was however the nasal equivalent of a voyeur in respect of his mistress' slippers and mittens). The novelist Adam Mars-Jones latches on to the oddity of smell in his memoir *Blind Bitter Happiness*—that it can be an almost universally unminded sense-faculty yet the one which offers the most empirically reliable discrimination—in the account of the car accident that left his mother Sheila without functioning olfactory nerves: 'Whether because the sensing fibres had been flattened by the van's impact, or because the area of the brain that interpreted their signals had been closed down while the blood pressure built up unnoticed, Sheila never smelt anything again, not fresh bread nor burning hair. The technical term for this is anosmia. Strange: loss of sight or hearing are privileged with an Anglo-Saxon term, while loss of smell remains in Greek, as if this is a rather fancy description. Never mind that smell is the most basic sense, the one that crouches lowest in the brain.'

Rachel Herz, a psychologist at Brown University, has shown that the gustatory and olfactive are faculties uniquely potent in evoking memory, having a direct connection with the hippocampus, a deep brain structure that seems to be the store of our longer-term memories. 'When from a long distant past nothing subsists,' wrote Marcel Proust, 'after the people are dead, after the things are broken and scattered, taste and smell alone [...] bear unflinchingly [...] the vast structure of recollection.' Herz found that smells produce emotionally intense recollections but not very intricate ones: they are association-poor. Lose your sense of smell, however, and nothing will ever taste quite the same.

Zoologically, smell is more prevalent among prosimians. Among Old World monkeys, catarrhines such as ourselves and the great apes rely on the much faster transmission of information imparted by visual and vocal signals. Olfactory cues, of less varied content perhaps but lingering and moving in all directions from the source, seem to be used for spacing and power relations, as well as to indicate sexual arousal. One great advantage of chemical signs is that they can signal in the absence of the individual who left the odour. In monkeys, smell is just one of several sexual cues, so that its lack can be compensated for by other means. Odour associations are learned by humans, and children exhibit no inherited reactions to smells. Despite this indifference to smell as a source of information, the smells we buy come in small but expensive bottles bearing the names of very large opera singers. They are designed to cover up our natural body odours. The French sage Michel de Montaigne suggested in his essay on smells: 'those fine foreign perfumes are rightly regarded as suspicious in those who use them; it may be thought that their purpose is to cover some natural defect in that quarter'. We seek to cover up our smells out of fear of eliciting disgust. And disgust, as the contemporary American social thinker William Ian Miller suggests in his pungent book *The Anatomy of Disgust*, allows us to moralise about other people with a clear conscience, especially under the conditions of modern civilised society: it is the cardinal moral sentiment. We are prompt to make value-judgements about people who use too much perfume, and those who don't use perfume at all. After all, scent 'is a brother of breath': it enters our very intimacy—deep through the limbic system—and there is little we can do to defend ourselves.

Things were different in the past. The Italian historian Piero Camporesi reminds us in his marvellous book about Italy in the middle ages, *Bread of Dreams*, a cornucopia of evocative nostrums and popular mythologies, that 'society of old was made up of a swarm of people, oiled, smeared, anointed and spiced, violently odorous and unbearably smelly, where everyone was in turn anointed and anointer, and where the sense of smell dominated heavily'. The French historian Alain Corbin has also published a great scholarly book about odours and the 'social imagination', *The Foul and the Fragrant*; it appeared a few years before the German novelist Patrick Süskind's remarkable debut novel, *Perfume*. Both books evoke the Paris of the early eighteenth century when the stench from the latrines and cesspools must have been so potent, imaginatively at least, that it hung around the streets until nineteenth-century couturiers and parfumiers, such as the House of Houbigant, found a way of making the grace-notes of plant-life—orange blossom, jasmine and honeysuckle—the essential adjunct to hedonism. Nosegays would slowly give way to aerosols.

By contrast, the primordial human effluvium, according to these books, is a sweaty-cheesy-oily stink. Observing the bowler-hatted inhabitants of the modern asphalt city around him in the 1920s, Bertolt Brecht was being anachronistic—but provocatively tolerant—when he wrote in his poem 'Of poor B.B.', 'They are quite particularly smelly animals. To which I say: it doesn't matter: so am I.'

V. S. Pritchett took the view that his fellow humans had, in the course of the same century, become markedly, and quite disappointingly, less odorous. In an essay written in 1980, he recalled the lusty aromas of London before the Great War. 'The smell of that London of my boyhood and bowler-hatted youth is still with me. The streets smelled of beer; men and boys reeked of hair oil, Vaseline, strong tobacco [...] The smell of women was racy and scented.' He had been captivated by what Jean-Jacques Rousseau would have called the search for the 'memorative sign', the collapsing of past into present when an odour is recognised which, far from leading into 'reverie', actually makes the self reveal its own affective history.

What is true is that humans are disgusted by strong smells now to a degree that wasn't the case a few hundred years ago. Once the civilizing process got going after Napoleon, and ours became a society of the spectacle, things changed for ever. And although we are all perfectly toilet-trained and no longer believe miasmas and vapours spell our doom, body odour still has a remarkable power to repulse and set apart, just in the same way that the festering foot-wound of the Greek hero Philoctetes got him isolated on an island on the campaign route to Troy. It wasn't so very long ago that the Nazis redefined the Jews as other-smelling. Disgust is so much more direct as a moral sentiment than hate, which needs *reasons*—all disgust needs is a whiff of body heat. What is as plain as the nose on anybody's face has often been an olfactory conviction first. For nothing arouses fear—and cancels pity—like a bad smell. As Freud suspected, smell is where desire and shame are compelled, within the contradictions of modern life, to have intercourse.

Even the German language, according to the once famous culture critic Ivan Illich, has lost nearly all its terms expressive of smell (although 'nose-wise'—*naseweis*—is a perfectly current German descriptive for a cheeky or precocious person). The Italian Bible scholar and essayist Guido Ceronetti is likewise adamant that the knowledge we have lost about the nose is knowledge we have lost about our selves: he insists—following Heraclitus—that souls smell things in Hades. He writes in his fascinating scrapbook on the history of medicine *The Silence of the Body*, 'The smelliest parts of the body are those where more soul is collected. The eye, which is odourless, is mirror not soul. Adding perfume to the body adds soul or allows people with no soul to pretend to have one. The strongest smells have come to disgust us, because the more civilisation represses and restrains natural animality, the more intolerable excessive soul becomes.' He also alludes to what he calls the sins of excessive cleanliness, Theresa of Avila's *limp-ieza demasiada*, and predicts that the squandering of our most basic resource—water—will take its revenge.

With his finely discriminatory nose, Nietzsche drew attention to himself as a geologist of concepts: he thought he was the only philosopher ever to get back to true basics. His war with the academy had started almost as soon as he was appointed to the chair of classical philology in Basel in 1869, aged twenty-four, and reached a peak with *The Genealogy of Morals*, his most decisive rejection of that unity of truth and reason expressed by the Encyclopedists. The genealogist requires a breaking up of flat assumptions so that radically new strata can emerge. Hence the importance of the nose. In the hierarchy of the senses, it is the sense most despised by reason, the most animalistic. Yet only a truly desperate man would want to claim that his genius was in his nostrils. In what were effectively his last sane words, Nietzsche was simultaneously reaching out into his own benightment and warning us, inadvertently perhaps, of reason's most subtle enemy, the subversive point of view that is everywhere. Nietzsche survived his own philosophy, and didn't know it. In the last instance, it was the nose—*his* nose—that was the best receptor for what he once called 'moraline', his scornful coining (it half-rhymes with nicotine) for the cloying perfumes of decomposition given off by those who think themselves virtuous.

With his desire to break out of the consummative idea of history that Christianity promulgated, and rediscover the endless cycles of India, Nietzsche would have appreciated the word *vasana*. 'It is the unknown that you should remember', the Jaiminiya Upanishad says; since the same lives appear and reappear over vast expanses of time, there can be nothing which corresponds to our concept of memory or recollection. Learning is reminding ourselves of what we have always known; and what triggers this reminding is *vasana*, or scent. This is the residue of a past life, which will be released only when a being is reincarnated in the same form. The nose allows everything to be a re-enactment.

Stendal's stories follow the logic of the epigram and anecdote, the remorselessness of logic itself: his art is one of codes and improvisations—'my passionate cohabitation with mathematics' he called it in *The Life of Henry Brulard*. In *The Privileges*, the short wish-list scribbled down as a kind of jocular testament in Rome two years before he died, he commanded 'The *corpus* and what comes out of it odourless.' The reek of the real wasn't something to detain Stendhal; lucidity was what he was after. Although sociability figures greatly in his work, it is a surface phenomenon. Not so Gogol. It was Nabokov who pointed out that the smells of the same Rome are implicated in the origins of Gogol's wonderful story of the disembodied truant nose: while he was travelling through Tuscany, the Ukrainian writer was almost preternaturally nose-conscious and wrote that the flowers of Italy gave him an overwhelming desire to be transformed into a Nose 'with nostrils the size of two goodly pails so that I might inhale all possible vernal perfumes'.

In must be a similar chemistry that excites the bored stationmaster on the Southern Austrian Railways in Joseph Roth's marvellous short story 'Fallmerayer the Stationmaster': he falls in love with a Russian countess who needs to recuperate briefly in his house after a train accident nearby; she leaves 'an inextinguishable trace of cuir de Russie and some nameless scent' floating around his bedroom. For months he lives in her 'sillage'—the train of scent left by a fragrant woman. Sent to fight on the Russian front in the Great War, he tracks down the countess and 'he smelt again the scent which for countless years had pursued him, which had surrounded, enclosed, tortured and consoled him'.

That is the special charisma of smell, and it has not escaped the notice of the modern perfume industry, which so generously tries to add zest to our lives of olfactory deprivation in the cities of numbed noses. Do we really need the perfume industry, though? Go outdoors on a windy April morning and you'll find yourself inhaling buckets of crisp vernal weather spiced with anemones as if assuaging some profound but barely describable yearning: as the Italian poet Giacomo Leopardi noted, the smell of something beautiful makes us want to merge with its source. That was surely what drew Dante to describe paradise itself—where God governs without intermediary and the laws of nature no longer apply—as a sempiternal yellow rose whose petals are the souls of the blessed. The praises ascending sunwards are the emanations of its perfume. And there is no windshadow, for all is radiance.

(Stendhal to Nikolai Vasilievich Gogol: if you want to get to heaven you'll have to leave your nose behind.)

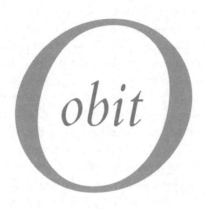

obit

The Importance of being an Agoraphobe

THE WRITINGS OF PETR SKRABANEK

Petr Skrabanek (1940–94) was one of the few really distinctive voices in post-war medicine: a polymath, world authority on substance P (a neurotransmitter) and Joyce scholar who ran yearly seminars on *Finnegans Wake*. He was on a visit to Yeats' grave in Sligo in 1968 when the Soviet army invaded Czechoslovakia. He and his future wife decided to stay in Ireland, and he completed his medical studies there in 1970. So began his mature career as 'natural scientist, forensic toxicologist, doctor of medicine and connoisseur of the absurd', and it culminated in an associate professorship at Trinity College. Skrabanek was a dissenter, fearless in his criticism of what he dubbed 'cacademics', 'quackupuncturists' and 'nonsensus-consensus'. The title of his best known book, *Follies and Fallacies in Medicine*, speaks for itself.

At last, someone has had the sense to bring out a selection of his several hundred published essays. This selection of sixteen of them gives a keen sense of the distinctive, witty manner in which he applied an 'attitude of mind rather than a philosophy': topics include electro-convulsive therapy, acupuncture, psychiatric nosology, anti-smoking campaigns and a brilliant Socratic dialogue defending 'destructive' criticism. ('All criticism welcome provided it is constructive', was the message I received from a journal editor the other day, in a perhaps only partly conscious attempt to defang criticism of its very *raison d'être*.) Skrabanek was anything but a rationalist by rote or bulk purchase. Overneat conceptual rationalisations are among his choice targets: Freud's and others' bespoke therapies write themselves off as science precisely because of their snap-shut snugness, the responsibility of the true scientist being to strive to find ways of proving himself wrong. 'By choosing unbelief', Skrabanek wrote in *False Premises, False Promises*, 'we do not rule out a subsequent change of opinion, based on new evidence, and thus nothing is lost; whereas, by being gullible, we lose reason from the very beginning.' Criticism is really the quickest way to learn. Whetted by Hume and Popper, his native wit is jugulating: 'Iconoclasm has no place in science because science has nothing to venerate.' Nor, he might have added, can its results be settled by plebiscite, or even by experts.

Medicine is a different matter, especially now that its methods of caring for the sick are overlaid with all sorts of socio-cultural agendas and quasi-religious expectations. It aspires to be a science though it is guided by notions of orthodoxy and heresy. As a social utility, it is ruled by conceptions of the *summum bonum* that are outside the remit of science: scientific method disregards issues of good and evil, indeed is successful as a method insofar as it does so, and therefore cannot be used as a moral guide. Unfortunately, doctors undergo a crammed, often dogmatic training in thrall to clinical 'bosses', which tends to hinder critical thinking. Then one fine day they wake up to find themselves as soteriological salesmen in the Valley of the Shadow of Death. And they hate to lose face by admitting they don't know. Honest ignorance, as Skrabanek insists, is preferable to dogma. Yet dogma is precisely what we have in mass screening and health checks—public health measures blessed by the global clergy of the Church of Happy and Merited Health (Geneva, not Rome).

One of Skrabanek's targets is epidemiology. Epidemiology— the branch of medicine that studies epidemics—used to be a minor discipline concerned with infectious diseases. Though such diseases have become markedly less prevalent, epidemiologists have not faded away; quite the reverse. The media of mass communication now serve as the best model for the spread of communicable diseases: sociogenic ones. 'The knowledge of risk factors rarely, if ever, contributes to the elucidation of causal mechanisms.' Many crucial associations continue to be made by clinical observation although the old-fashioned case report (a testimony about the natural history of a disease in an individual patient) has lost nearly all the prestige it once enjoyed in medical journals: it is ranked lowest in the evidence hierarchy of current biomedical research. Skrabanek mentions the now-forgotten study in the 1980s that seemed to show that AIDS was causally related to the use of 'poppers' (amyl nitrite): such is the complexity of association in the real world that the very method of analysing and reporting data may itself construct or confound certain 'findings', and be quite unrelated to cause. This applies particularly to low-level risks.

Skrabanek called this kind of associationist epidemiology 'black box thinking'. The 'black box' is an untested postulate which strives to link exposure and disease. In practice, it means looking at, say, a cause of mortality and then sifting populations for differences in death rates so as to determine *ex post hoc* the principal causes of mortality. An association, by definition a fortuitous finding, is thus magicked retrospectively into a causal link. No smoke without fire, the public is invited to think, although Hume long ago made cause and effect far more problematic notions than they might seem. Kant summed up the Scottish philosopher's scepticism thus: 'he inferred that Reason completely deceives herself with this concept, in falsely taking it for her own child, whereas it is nothing but a bastard of the imagination fathered by experience'. As a man of good sense, Hume merely observed that without access to the deeper causes of things we ought not to mistake our value judgements for absolute truths: an accumulation of facts is not sufficient to establish a universal law. But it seems to be characteristic of our age that a loose association of ideas is commonly mistaken for a solid argument. These associational factors are then regarded as the intellectual equivalent of socially threatening Dickensian imps and urchins: a regulating bureaucracy is called for; public information, enquiries and watchdogs, outcome measurements, more bureaucracy, and so on. More than three hundred 'risk-markers' have been identified for coronary heart disease, and the list keeps lengthening. If we have to have lists, why not go back to the nine rigorous criteria drawn up by Sir Austin Bradford Hill in 1965, which ought to be considered in any attempt to ascribe cause? They were strength, consistency, specificity, plausibility, coherence, biological gradient, experimental evidence, temporality and analogy—only the last two carry any weight with the media and public. Indeed, scare stories are topical analogies that have run riot.

The practical effect of Skrabanek's concern is best seen in his 1990 essay 'Why is Preventive Medicine Exempted from Ethical Constraints?' Early preventive medicine grew out of hygiene and medical policing, which involved treating some people (on behalf of the state) as if they were weeds in a flourishing market garden. Some preventive measures such as vaccination have a clear benefit but others do not, and their mass deployment results in labelling, anxiety and medicalisation. While medical experiments on individuals have been subject, since 1947, to the need to obtain fully informed consent, screening campaigns got going among the populations of most developed countries with almost no prior discussion of what outcomes might reasonably be expected. Prevention is always better than cure, isn't it? 'The issues of preventive medicine have little to do with science, relative risks, and risk factors. They could be more profitably debated within the framework to which they belong—ethics, politics, and vested interests.' It might be more honest to call them population experiments or forms of early diagnosis. Certainly they fuel what sociologists call the 'ecological fallacy'—the presumption that individual destiny can be modified on the basis of evidence gathered from the study of populations. Significantly, as medicine proceeds towards a disaster of good intention (a controversial review in The Lancet at the start of 2000 suggested screening for breast cancer does not reduce mortality), it has come to rely increasingly on consensus conferences. Good science has no need for consensus, Skrabanek dryly remarks, since consensus is an essentially political notion, and a crying need for it arises only in its absence. Yet it was a politician (Nye Bevan) who, at the outset of the National Health Service, quoted Galileo's warning about mistaking the methods of science for what they are they not: 'The aim of science is not to open a door on infinite wisdom, but to set a limit to infinite error.'

Those sharp-eyed nineteenth-century French social observers Tocqueville and Constant noted—especially in consideration of the budding United States—that the desire for well-being might push democracies to surrender their liberty, perhaps without fully realising it. Skrabanek grew up in a totalitarian society based on the idea of the perfectibility of man; and it is surely his traditional Czech respect for a clear philosophical head that makes him insist that life will always be elsewhere for those who believe happiness can be defined bureaucratically, as a health plan. A similar conceptual boldness and disdain for prescription-writers can be heard in the essays of his countryman, the late Miroslav Holub, who was an immunologist and poet of world rank. One of Holub's caustic remarks about the supposed 'wisdom' of crowds (a trendy topic these days) reflects Skrabanek's experience too: 'stupidity multiplies in a herd, whereas reason is divided by the number of heads, and reason thus diminishes with multitude'. To be subversive is to think in the face of fear, especially when the herd publicly gangs up on you. Anyone who has anything to do with the health sciences will profit greatly from Skrabanek's book: it will loosen them from the bonds of what W. H. Auden memorably called 'infernal science', or what even the ruthless Francis Bacon, in the first days of materialism as matter and mode of investigation, considered *idola fori*—idols of the market.

It is sobering to think that the practical effort required for 'the relief of man's estate', as Bacon called it, might just as comprehensively relieve man of his estate.

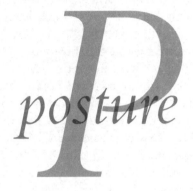

posture

The Human Position

ON FLYING AND FALLING

1

In the waiting room of my surgery in Strasbourg there are a number of paintings and etchings. These have been loaned to me by my landlord, who is one of the city's elder artists (Philippe Stoll-Litschgy). I suppose having his work on the walls lends a certain chic appeal to my surgery, but it sometimes makes me a little nervous to think that I'm curator of an art gallery in addition to having to attend to the humdrum of running a medical practice. But these paintings have another function: they allow me to stand in my waiting room and daydream in broad daylight, surrounded by mythic themes: I extend invitations to all and sundry, I offer my card—here I am, dear townspeople of Strasbourg: come and watch how to fly away from uncertainty.

One of the works on the wall is a woodcut showing Icarus with two improbable retaining bands tied to his ankles as he plummets earthwards in a squawk of quill feathers. Unlike Brueghel's painting and W. H. Auden's commentary on it, Icarus' fall rearranges the landscape; the objects in the woodcut form a spatial choir around it. A nymph shields her eyes. An elephant does something elephantine. The leaves shiver. It is a cinematic moment where agent, matter and observer are the three separate dimensions of a boy-angel's body which has entered time the wrong way. Sadly, nobody can now explain to Icarus the persistent flaw in the story of his pratfall since if he really had decided to fly high when his father said he shouldn't, then the higher he flew the cooler and less resistant the ambient air would have been: wax or no wax, trailing edges at height become more efficient.

The etching made me go back to Auden's famous poem about Icarus, which he wrote in Brussels in December 1938, just a month before he made his own flight from a Europe on the edge of war to the haven of the United States. It dilates laconically on one of the great myths of knowledge (in some ways a mirror-image of the Oedipus myth); Icarus flutters out of an upstairs Cretan window and shimmers peculiarly and incandescently across our technological age, the age of bombing. Auden called his poem 'Musée des Beaux Arts' after the gallery where he saw the painting in Brussels:

> About suffering they were never wrong,
> The Old Masters: how well they understood
> Its human position...

Suffering happens, and other things happen too: someone eats an apple or a pear, or opens the window to air the house, or just strolls empty-headedly past. Dogs get on with their doggy lives, and 'the torturer's horse' rubs its rump on a tree. With his fleeting references to Pieter Brueghel's masterly studies of terror, 'The Numbering at Bethlehem' and 'The Slaughter of the Innocents', Auden then turns his attention to 'Landscape with the Fall of Icarus' (1588), in which all that can be seen of Icarus is a pair of flailing legs about to disappear beneath the surface of the water.

>   how everything turns away
> Quite leisurely from the disaster: the ploughman may
> Have heard the splash, the forsaken cry,
> But for him it was not an important failure...

Icarus looks like a flying trickster who hasn't quite perfected his water entry technique, one of those medieval airmen who regularly used to launch themselves from battlements and fortifications to sudden death or, if they survived coming a cropper, like Father Damian, the fifteenth-century Italian-born Scotsman who tried to fly with feathered wings from Stirling Castle to Paris, to the slower death of public derision: Father Damian broke both his legs in the castle moat. In the foreground of Brueghel's painting a ploughman cuts a furrow in a clay field whose furrows run to the edge of the field of vision: it is an image redolent of inertia, custom and tradition. The ship is of a kind Brueghel would have seen anywhere off the coast of the Low Countries: it floats on the aquatic beatitude of a world newly made by money. The Dutch were rapidly expanding as the foremost maritime power: 1588 was the year that a fierce gale in the English Channel destroyed the redoubtable Spanish Armada. Not included in Auden's poem is a fisherman on the bank who seems oblivious to what's going on around him, and a shepherd who, perhaps hearing something—a creak, a cry—, is leaning on his staff and looking skywards, though in the wrong direction altogether. In a thicket close to the border of the painting—even less apparent than the drowning Icarus—lies the bald head of an unburied corpse, face up. Away in the distance a fabulous red-roofed city shimmers in the early light.

The very moment Icarus comes into view he drops out of it altogether.

The painting tugs at custom and fable in a way the poem does not: art historians tell us that although his source was Book 8 of Ovid's *Metamorphoses*, Brueghel's intention was to actualise the harsh popular Flemish saying, 'No plough comes to a standstill for a dying man.' Auden makes mundanity the bearer of understanding, but permits only the Old Masters (something he was to become himself in his poet's progress) the cosmic amusement: to *have* the understanding. The morally critical incident, Icarus' slippage, is of passing relevance, and his fall happens practically *hors scène*. Auden's pronouns are evasive too: to what does the 'it' refer, for instance, in the opening lines? In this Arcadian costume drama humans are surrounded by a surfeit of gerunds: suffering, eating, opening, walking, waiting, skating, disappearing, falling—none of them is able to follow the action through to completion. His voice in this poem is seductively reasonable and commonsensical: that is why we should distrust it, since common sense may also be an open trap.

So what *is* the 'human position' of suffering? Why make this idea explicit when the painting instructs the dead to bury their own?

Icarus' fall may be spectacular, but it's not evident why it should be thought of as giving access to the quality of suffering. Icarus, like the subject in one of the most vertiginous of all Futurist paintings, Tullio Crali's *Incuneandosi nell'abitato* (Nose-diving on a City, 1939), which shows the cockpit view from behind a pilot as he plummets vertically down on a circuit board of skyscrapers, is man on the move, rushing into his death. What happens next is forgotten in the vertigo of the image. Suffering, Auden's poem suggests by contrast, is not something exceptional or dramatic: commonplace, uncharismatic, it may be as near as the next life and yet utterly remote. There is nothing subtle about it. When the dying Mrs Gradgrind in Dickens' *Hard Times* is asked: 'Are you in pain, dear?', and she replies, 'There is a pain somewhere in the room, but I cannot be positive that I've got it', her reply makes no phenomenological sense at all, for pain leaves no room at all for doubt. Pain is a state of being that impales us solipsists on the sensation of time itself. It is one of the great stubborn facts of existence, a quality we can't deny in ourselves but, equally, can't confirm in others. In terms of cognition, it reinforces the bounds of privacy, while undermining everything solid about others; in terms of recognition, it stakes its claims outside the field of knowledge altogether. The demand for *acknowledgement* is pain's social life.

In another sense pain is the invisible, subterranean geography that swallows up Icarus' head. (Wittgenstein couldn't understand how pain could have *depth*, although it's only paint-deep in our example). For a person of Auden's generation, it's easy to see that geography as the trenches of the First War. Nothing about the nature of war would ever be the same again: people begin to be seen in terms of mass, mud is the medium, and hard steel strips the tiny, vulnerable human frame of whatever pathetically inadequate dignity it has left. Brute matter remains itself, but the shell shock goes deep into language.

In 1909, just a few years before the war made the connection between flight and alienation explicit, and decades before Europe was an afterglow of burning cities, Kafka wrote in his diary, having just attended an aviation meeting in Brescia, 'What is happening? Here above us, there is a man twenty metres above the earth, imprisoned in a wooden frame, and defending himself against an invisible danger which he has taken on of his own free will. But we are standing below, pushed away, without existence, and looking at this man.' Aeroplanes? 'Upchartered choristers of their own speeding', was how the American poet Hart Crane dubbed them.

Or we can go back, but only through museum glass, to the original state of innocence in which winged flight and bombing (the first aerial bombardment actually took place in 1849) were anticipated by Leonardo da Vinci when he designed his orni-thopter; man was to ascend into the air 'in order to look for snow on the mountain tops, and then return to scatter it over the city streets shimmering with the heat of summer'.

2

But let me return instead to the semantic energies of the poem: notice how Auden concentrates our attention on the peculiarly active sense of what '*takes* place' in the poem. The verb seems to engulf its sentence, to be a species of rhetorical hygiene.

No one would dispute that suffering is the unbearable index of our uniqueness: part of the way it provokes a turning away in those who witness it is its resistance to language. What materiality it has is mute. The distress and embarrassment we often feel in front of the suffering of others comes about because we don't know what to say. Consolation may seem an upsurge too easily bought by words. Pain itself destroys language, or at least reduces sustained utterance to cries and whimpers, animal beseechings. To put it another way, sentient hurt has no object, and people are obliged to find parallels for it: 'Doctor, it feels as if...'. This is what the doctor himself is supposed to speak for, as the patient's advo-cate or intermediary; and the doctor's surgery should be the one place a patient can be sure the reality of his suffering is acknowl-edged and given terms of reference. In practice, expressing pain is a prelude to its alleviation, and nobody should ever think reality betrayed by that one welling moment of imaginative empathy.

What irritates me about the poem, since I recognise its temptations and deferments, and can feel even as I write what it means to want to escape, is the resignation to the lamentational mode in the absolutism of the phrase 'they were never wrong'. Nietzsche, a psychologist every bit as perspicuous as Auden, once wrote, 'I've given a name to my pain and call it "dog"', which wins assent, since it evinces a kind of courage. It is theatrical. We know, as Nietzsche did, the ultimate hopelessness of the cause. Whipped, shouted at, or fetching metaphysical bones, pain-as-dog is company.

But as my adjective 'theatrical' hints, pain has entered another dimension: that of *performance*. Writers, as a genus, have little difficulty performing. The trouble generally with suffering in the Musée is that artists represent suffering so well and make it so convincingly visible that they come to be thought of as the most authentically suffering group of individuals. This is how Kafka, with his unnervingly acute way of formulating a dilemma (it is one first voiced by Edgar in King Lear: 'The worst is not / So long as we can say, 'This is the worst.'') confides in his diary: 'Have never understood how it is possible for almost everyone who writes to objectify his sufferings in the very thick of them: I, for example, in the midst of my unhappiness, in all likelihood with my head still smarting from unhappiness, sit down and write to someone: I am unhappy. Yes, I can even go beyond that and with as many embellishments as I have talent for, all of which seem to have nothing to do with my unhappiness, ring simple, or contrapuntal, or a whole orchestration of changes on my theme. And it is not a lie, and it does not quiet my pain; it is simply a merciful surplus of strength at a moment when suffering has raked me to the bottom of my being and plainly exhausted all my strength. But then what kind of surplus is it?'

Kafka rightly felt that there was something dubious about being a writer. This feeling bothered Auden in mid-life too; his cleverness in introducing a torturer's horse and martyrdom to the scene show at least how the failure to express pain can be co-opted, not so much to extend culture, but to break it up. The bystanders' disinterest in Icarus' thwarted but armourless flight seems to be a projection of the airman's detachment from the mass observation subjects obliterated on the ground below. Auden understands the situation like a neuro-psychiatrist: consciousness is a shield protecting us *against* experience. Self puts on its conscious life as if it were a steel helmet in order to block the impress of so much sensory bombardment, from the subatomic to the Icarian. To survive, we have to cheat ourselves of experience. Or, to put it another way: if we intend to be judges we dare not feel too acutely the reality of what we judge.

Many psychoanalytically minded critics have been tempted to read 'Musée des Beaux Arts' as if it were autobiography—a kind of confession. It suggests a map of Auden's own feelings after having urged his social imaginary to stand up and be counted in the fight against fascism, only to renounce political engagement by leaving for the United States. Icarus, after all, has just failed to fly away from the labyrinth—from art. In 'Voltaire at Ferney', another poem written at that time, Auden provides a reassessment of the same crisis—'all over Europe stood the horrible nurses / Itching to boil their children'—an image from an empire on its way down, and one which startles because a public schoolboy's nightmare seems so grotesquely inadequate to the hard rain that Auden all through the thirties had said was coming. His conclusion to this poem harks back to the quite leisurely turning away of the Icarus poem: 'The uncomplaining stars composed their lucid song.' Evoking the stars—so far above us we can't covet them, as Goethe said—advertises the triumph of pain; the song might be lucid, but its cadence isn't human. Star-gazing isn't something we should do alone. Indeed, for Walter Benjamin, the recently finished war had been 'an attempt at new and unprecedented commingling with the cosmic powers. Human multitudes, gases, electrical forces were hurled into open country, high-frequency currents coursed through the landscape, new constellations rose in the sky, aerial space and ocean depths thundered with propellers, and everywhere sacrificial shafts were dug into Mother Earth.'

With his fine instinct for personal existential choice and disregard for the logic of his own position, it looks as if dear old Auden had decided to reach down for his slippers in the famous chaotic life of books in Middagh Street, Brooklyn, and adopt the American avuncular of Uncle Whiz. His decision to quit Britain at its worst moment still causes rancour (it has been said that he 'defected' like his friend Guy Burgess), usually followed by the insinuation that in so doing he not only lost touch with his natural constituency of readers but with the mother-tongue. One American writer, Guy Davenport, commented: 'he wanted a place he could not romanticize. He came [to New York] to ensure that he was among humanity at its worst in this century.' Well, that's saying it for America! It sounds like an act of self-mortification. Auden was courageous in that he refused to be bullied by ancestral claims ('because I knew then that if I stayed, I would inevitably become a member of the British establishment') or even to acknowledge the contingent impersonal claims of history. His move to the States marks a crisis in his own search for the good life: a genuine allegiance to the political and moral community in which he had grown up would have made the nature of his political obligation obvious to him—there would have been no choice to make. He *renounced* his past in order to suffer the wrong life. Estrangement was the neurosis he chose to cultivate. It is not that he lost touch with his language; it is rather than he was obliged, by his act, to scrutinise what it meant to be a moral hero; more particularly, what it meant to *want* to be a moral hero in a democratic age.

3

And Daedalus? Daedalus ('the ingenious') is always absent from these pictures. Either he's picking up the feathers of his archaic flying machine scattered on the surface of the sea, or he's back in the workshop on Kill Devil Hill going over and over the drag coefficient of his flyer, correcting his notes on the mathematics of birdflight as a basis for aviation. He doesn't know any other way to be a father. His legs tremble, he can barely hold himself erect for grief. Now he feels the full force of not being able to take his son's place, and fall in his stead. He clutches the sink, vomiting out his son's quip about 'climbing up to oneself by climbing above oneself' (Nietzsche). Perhaps he blames himself for passing on the technology before the boy was ready for it: his time register was always horizontal, empirical, strenuous, never the plummet of now his son flirted with. 'Profundum, physical thunder, dimension in which / We believe without belief, beyond belief', was how Wallace Stevens called it in his little squib *Flyer's*

Fall. Gottfried Benn's Icarus poem of 1915 is the most extreme expression of this regressive urge to 'bloom to death', not so much a sublime attempt to fuse with the solid world below—or to merge with the divine mind, like Goethe's Ganymede—but a wild urge to plummet out of consciousness altogether and down through the phylogenetically old pathways of the brainstem—spinoretic-ular, palaeospinothalamic and propriospinal, as they were termed before Benn attended medical school—to a flinty, inorganic *terra incognita* where his left frontal lobe (Broca's area) somehow still functions:

> Still through the scree on the foothills, still through
> > land-carrion,
> turning to dust, through beggarly jagged
> cliff-edges—everywhere
> deep mother-blood, this streaming
> decerebrate
> slack
> wearing away.

Daedalus is a bit of a fogey: he represents knowledge as baggage—it gives him ballast, keeps him ponderous and methodical, but gets him home. His is the awful I-saw-it-coming condescension of posterity. His warnings to his son not to go off on his own course, not to swoop too low and wet his wings or soar too high and blaze out in one final moment of white heat—this warning is the clearest indication that Daedalus has read his son's mind, that he knows every intricate dimension of his son's secret wish to overreach him long before he had even thought of those wings, as Miroslav Holub, the Czech immunologist and poet noted in his poem *On Daedalus*, which swarms with Icaruses:

> In the airport lounge (automatic goodbyes);
> at the space control centre (transistorised metempsychosis).
> on the sports ground (enrolment of pupils born 1970),
> in the museum (blond seepage of beards),
> on the ceiling (a rainbow stain of imagination);
> in the swamps (hooting of night, born 1640);
> in the stone (Pleistocene finger pointing upwards).

For a man who was to invent the steam-bath, the reservoir, glue, the plumbline and the axe, Daedalus should have been able to foresee almost anything. Father and son were fleeing from the labyrinth Daedalus had earlier devised for King Minos on Crete. The king had imprisoned them both in fury after Daedalus had helped one of Poseidon's white bulls to copulate with King Minos' wife Pasiphae, the union resulting in the Minotaur, that hybrid of man, beast and jousting machine that was to become the maze's monster attraction until the arrival of Theseus. Mutants and labyrinths lurk where the lust for knowledge, *libido sciendi*, meets up with human ingenuity. Or as Ovid reasons, in a famous couplet about the bull-man, man-bull: *Daedalus ut clausit conceptum crimine matris / Semibouemque uirum semiuirumque bouem...*

4

Why was Daedalus exiled on Crete at all? Because he had earlier pushed his own nephew and apprentice Talos off the Acropolis; Talos' ingenuity as a craftsman in his own right (inventor of the saw, compass and potter's wheel) had been threatening to obscure Daedalus' considerable fame. Talos was changed into a partridge, a bird that lost its head for heights while saving its skin, as in Michael Longley's poem *Perdix*:

> a grim reminder to Daedalus
> —Inventor, failure's father—of his apprentice, a boy
> Who had as a twelve-year-old the mental capacity
> To look at the backbone of a fish and invent the saw
> By cutting teeth in a metal blade [...]

And when his talented apprentice 'slips' off the edge of a rockface at the Acropolis, Daedalus is economical with the truth,

> but Pallas Athene
> Who supports the ingenious, intercepted his fall,
> Dressed him in feathers in mid-air and made him a bird...

Not much scientific dispassion there. Clearly their apprentice-master relationship was lacking in the kind of strictures and structures which are common to every vocation in modern times and which might have helped to avoid the later retributive business with Icarus. For example, some of the tough inflexible professional strictures that medical students put up with and eventually aspire to enter: strictly determined professional status, knowledge acquisition as ordeal, solemn rites of passage, critical appraisal by peers. The titles of some of Auden's favourite books in the thirties suggest just the interest he took in some of those loyalty-binding shibboleths, as set out in John Layard's *Degree-Taking Rites in the South West Bay of Malekula*. Those are the trappings, after all, that protect future doctors from indecent exposure to pity.

Knowledge decays. Daedalus was in a rut in Crete, despite all the ingenuity he had devoted to developing the world's first artificial insemination technique for cross-species hybridisation. Perhaps it's a mistake to practise sex therapy on kings' wives. Nevertheless he chose to take the baggage along with him, all those rusty old ideas, their built-in obsolescence, the past's colossal burden. That is perhaps why Socrates liked to claim descent from Daedalus. His knowledge was intellectual skill, artisanal and applied; it was rooted in the real world. He might have been the kind of doctor who invents and patents ergonomically efficient surgical instruments: the father of Denis Diderot perhaps, who, in his master cutler's workshop in Langres, produced surgical lancets of such high quality they were bought all over France and put to even greater use, at least metaphorically, by his son. He would have marvelled at the great flying cathedrals of our age: the 165 tons, six million parts, twenty-one thousand horse-power thrust of a Boeing 747. The insinuation that flight was an escape from one's proper business would have baffled him.

Time is full of Icaruses: if a son symbolises anything to his father, then Icarus was the sweep of progress, the high of pure theory, the flight from authority, the quick fix of the new—'Zarathustra the dancer, Zarathustra the light, he who beckons with his wings, poised to fly, beckoning to all the birds, poised and ready, blessed in the ease of his levity.' Icarus thought he could gull his old man and came down with his engines on fire. It wasn't the sun that scorched his wings; in his father's language, he was actually the first case of professional burn-out: his waxy quill wings flared in the wind, torched from the *inside*, and down he fell, not on a bed of humbled assumptions but on the hard ground rising.

5

This is why those few curious people who venture into my surgery are compelled to think of Icarus, a less complex and interesting figure than Daedalus (the Dent compendium *Who's Who in Classical Mythology* gets it right with its caption heading 'Icarus: *see* DAEDALUS'): the symbol of the age is something as inherently unstable as man trying to fly by travelling light, incorrigible and alone. Icarus is a fictional extreme—that is why he is so easy to represent. The real problem for the bystander, though, as he fills his head with more and more about less and less, and as knowledge reduces its half-life, is to determine whether he more closely resembles Daedalus the anaesthetist, or Icarus the air-head. Technical civilisation offers him a fantasy of total bodily comfort—its underside is a shattered body politic where he can replay other people's catastrophes all day long. In our electronic ether, proximate electromagnetic pain is a thought away and we all have some quotient in what Ernst Jünger called the 'Second Consciousness', the statistical probability in war and peace (that is to say the moral irresponsibility) of becoming a technological casualty like Icarus. But it was Jünger who, throughout the 1920s and most spectacularly in his influential book *Storm of Steel*, aimed to repudiate Benjamin's recognition of just how tiny and vulnerable the human body knew itself to be, opting instead for a kind of armoured perception, a full metal jacket for those who, like himself, were fascinated by the spectacle of mythic horror rearing up in the middle of a civilisation of gleaming steel. If Jünger cultivated an observational coldness, other ideologies of hardness would serve the functionalism of the Nazi state.

If Icarus' fate is an allegory of self-delusion, the punishable conduct of a son who had yet to hear about Oedipus, his father by contrast seems both disciplined against and vulnerable to the shock of history. The historicist humbles himself by admitting his own historicism. Or as Auden put it, poets have to be tough to maintain their fragility, which is to say that the qualities that allow them to be most productive are also their Achilles' heel.

6

Now, as I wait for patients, I steal a glance out the window and suspect I resemble Icarus, who probably didn't have the perseverance and staying power to become a Daedalus. And now that Auden, (in my heretical opinion) a more convincing essayist than he was a poet, has himself has become a whole climate of opinion, I'd like to ask his gentle ghost one more thing: what would an Old Master 'understand' of those who can't turn away?

My position, for the time being, is firmly on my gluteals, which is just as well since, as Michel de Montaigne—who loved nothing more than to be seated on his horse—observed, 'even on the highest throne in the world we only ever sit on our own rump'. Too much abstraction leads to a craving for the concrete, any old concrete.

The sedentary station doesn't stop me from feeling weightless though, especially now that I notice I don't have any patients.

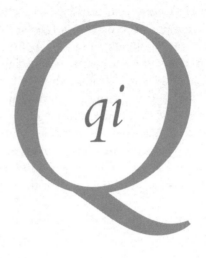

Emergent properties

JOSEPH NEEDHAM AND CHINA

One of the great synoptic works of developmental biology is a three-volume set published by Cambridge University Press in 1931. I heard about this book when I studied developmental biology myself, halfway through my medical degree; and the professor of anatomy under whom I studied had nothing but praise for its author. Over two thousand pages long, *Chemical Embryology* provides not only an exhaustive account of physiological changes in the embryo and placenta (osmotic pressure, pH, respiratory gradients, metabolic processes) but a descriptive history of the egg from its earliest mythic beginnings. 'Practically nothing was left out', wrote its author—one Joseph Needham, born 1900, only son of a Harley Street physician specialising in anaesthetics and an erratic, high-strung mother (who so seldom saw eye to eye with her husband that she called her son by a different Christian name). Leading light of the Cambridge Biochemical Laboratory, he was already being hailed as the new Erasmus, so impressive were his intellectual reach and vigour. He did have the benefits of a photographic memory. His wife Dorothy—'Dophi'—Moyle, herself a noted biochemist, recalled him lying awake in bed, energised by the work he had been doing in the hours before—'mentally visualising the book's page proofs, and then correcting in a notebook any errors or infelicities'.

Needham liked bringing things between covers, and it wasn't always writings on biology. Wayward driver of an Armstrong-Siddeley Tourer, brazen gymnosophist (nude bather), radical activist, forbearing Anglo-Catholic and keen morris dancer, he was also acquiring a considerable reputation as a skirt-chaser. To be an eccentric in Cambridge went with the turf; to be unsound was to invite social ostracism. But Needham knew just how to toe the line, and people would make allowances for him because of his brilliance. Then in 1936, three Chinese research assistants came to work in his lab. He began a relationship with the female member of the team, Lu Gwei-djen, a physiologist from Nanjing, who stayed on in Cambridge: their affair was to last, with the complaisance of Dophi, for the next half-century. All three must have spent many a jolly evening together in the local pub discussing the biomechanics of muscle tissue.

Theirs was to be a significant encounter in another way. Lighting a post-coital Player's for her one evening in 1938, Needham casually asked her how 'cigarette' would be written in Mandarin. Lu Gwei-djen guided his hand, inscribing the ideogram that seemed far more poetic in literal translation than the English word: *fragrant smoke*. A cigarette had been the catalyst: 'I must learn this language—or bust!' he told her. Within a couple of years Needham had produced a series of homemade notebooks detailing 6000 characters indexed in terms of their radicals and cross-referenced to English words. The task of learning Chinese made him, in his own words, 'almost delirious with happiness'. (He was still spending his days as a biochemist.)

With the war in its third year, and large parts of China under Japanese control, a member of the Royal Society (of which Needham was now a fellow) suggested that a senior figure connected with British research should be airlifted into China, as head of a new body with quasi-diplomatic status to be called the Sino-British Scientific Cooperation Office (SBSCO). Needham was the obvious choice. His duties were to include organising help for Chinese scholars fleeing the Japanese invaders, who were advancing into the inner provinces. Equipped with a Webley service revolver and diplomatic papers, he was flown in February 1943 into China over the notorious Hump, the airbridge that led east of Calcutta and across Burma to occupied China. He had just seen his second major work through the press, *Biology and Morphogenesis* (1942). His base was to be Chongqing, the capital of unoccupied China, at the humid confluence of the Yangzi and the Jialing: it is now said to be the world's most rapidly expanding city with a population of over thirty-five million.

It was a dangerous mission, full of hair-raising logistical difficulties, but Needham had a genius for improvisation and an 'imperturbable persistence'. The scholarly Grand Panjandrum had derring-do, and Simon Winchester devotes nearly half of his companionable biography to the three years in China. Needham was hardly ever in his office in Chongqing. He made no fewer than eleven sorties on behalf of the SBSCO, some of them fact-gathering missions but others epic undertakings that were risky and, in one case—which involved crossing the frontline south-west to Fuzhou—'downright foolhardy'. The most spectacular of them all—his own Long March—involved driving two Chevrolet trucks northwards to what was then known as Chinese Turkestan. This trip allowed him to inspect the irrigation project set up at Dujiangyan in 250 BC on the orders of Li Bing, governor of the province, when water engineering first proved to be crucial to the welfare of the imperial system. His discovery that the water-works were still in working order brought him to a pitch of high excitement. Two months later they reached the Mogao Caves at Dunhuang, a Silk Road oasis on the edge of the western Gobi Desert and the repository of the world's oldest printed book, the Diamond Sutra, and thousands of other rare scrolls. The man who had actually found the library in 1907 and inspired Needham to make the trip, the famous explorer Sir Aurel Stein, was, unbeknown to Needham, actually lying on his death-bed just a few hundred miles away in Kabul.

When he left China in 1946, Needham had visited 296 Chinese institutes and universities. He helped lay the foundations for organisations to support Chinese science. It was not the only organisation he helped to establish: he was the administrator in Paris who, as his admirers later said, 'put the "s" into Unesco' as the founder and first director of its Natural Sciences section. Two years later, glad to be back at his rooms in Gonville and Caius, he began opening the hundreds of boxes and crates he had sent back to his college during the war. For daily work he now donned the traditional scholar's gown of blue silk he had acquired on his travels. In 1948 he addressed a proposal to the Syndics of Cambridge University Press: it was the outline of the work which would make him famous: *Science and Civilisation in China*.

In spite of a few querulous souls at the press who felt Needham ought to be doing what he was ostensibly there to do—teaching embryology and doing experimental work into the chemistry of early life (specifically inisotol levels in the chicken embryo)—he was given leave of teaching duties. From then on he was able, with the help of his assistant, the Chinese historian Wang Ling, to 'follow [his] star without distraction'. This is all the more remarkable when it is borne in mind that Needham had no academic standing in the actual department of Oriental Studies. Soon, some of the discoveries he had made in China—on the abacus, dam-making and plum-grafting techniques—were being supplemented by the results of methodical reading and judicious probing of Chinese sources. Needham had already been awarded one of the Republic's highest honours, but he had close ties with the new rulers too. In fact, he was so close to Zhou Enlai, Mao's foreign minister, as to be blind to the nature of the new regime: the Patriotic Hygiene Campaign under the Communists would, he believed, be China's saving. Loyalty to the Communists led Needham to put his entire career in jeopardy: in 1952 he took part in a Chinese-led inquiry into alleged use of germ warfare by the Americans during the Korean War. Hoaxed (it would appear) by a Soviet-inspired disinformation campaign, the inquiry's findings accused the Americans of dropping cholera-infected rats on northern villages. The entire British establishment, including parliament, the Royal Society and his own college, vented its fury on him—'some people called him a dupe, others a traitor, a few simply a crank'. And most inconveniently for his career, the State Department in the US blacklisted him until well into the 1970s. Like a long list of British intellectuals he had been naïve enough to think that politics worked on the same impartial principles as science. Where intentions were good acts would be good too.

Ending up *persona non grata* saved him for his work. Needham had read enough to start writing. Seven volumes were initially planned, of which the fifth would be devoted to what has since become known, even in Mandarin, as the Needham question (*Li Yuese nanti*): if the Chinese had been so technologically inventive, why did they not come up with modern science? 'Sci[ience] in general in China—why [did it] not develop?' was the original entry in his notebook. Wherever Needham looked the Chinese had been there first: fitting stirrups, steering with compasses, casting iron, inoculating against smallpox, recognising beri-beri, distilling mercury, making maps, ball-bearings, umbrellas and clockwork escapements… Yet just at the time when the Renaissance was in full flow in Europe the creative passions of the Celestial Kingdom were drying up. Needham was unsure. Perhaps his question was back-to-front: perhaps it ought to be 'why Europe (of all places)?' Was it related to mathematics, capitalism, or the peculiar 'doubleness' of the European mind and its fondness for viewing things as particles? It was a mind that was 'oscillating for ever unhappily between the heavenly host on one side and the "atoms and the void" on the other; while the Chinese, wise before their time, worked out an organic theory of the universe that included Nature and man, church and the state, and all things past, present and to come. It may well be that here, at this point of tension, lies some of the secret of the specific European creativeness when the time was ripe.' The question is still open.

When the first volume, *Introductory Orientations,* appeared in 1954, it was an immediate critical success. Even Needham's bitterest enemies praised it without stint: Laurence Picken, another Cambridge recruit to the SBSCO who had fallen out badly with him in Chongqing and was quite as brilliant a polymath (cytology, languages and ethnomusicology were his principal interests), wrote in the Manchester Guardian that its achievement was 'prodigious… perhaps the greatest single act of historical synthesis and intercultural communication ever attempted by one man'. The initial print-run sold out, and it has been reprinted several times since. When the second volume *History of Scientific Thought* appeared two years later, it was apparent to everybody that Needham's magnum opus was going to be something very remarkable indeed. Literary voices joined in the chorus of praise. George Steiner, no slouch himself, wrote that *Science and Civilisation in China* was the modern work that came closest to Marcel Proust's fictional attempt to recreate an entire society and past. He thought Needham was sympathetically reconstituting a prospect of the imagination forgotten by Chinese scholars themselves: 'Proust on the altering focus of the steeple at Martinville and Needham on man's realisation, across centuries and cultures, of the true shape of the snow crystal are exactly comparable exercises in total imaginative penetration. In each there is an intense poetry of thought, readily felt but extremely difficult to paraphrase.' It was in a little tractate, 'Strena, seu de Nive Sexangula' ('A New Year's Gift of Hexagonal Snow'), gifted to his patron Wackher von Wackenfels on New Year's Day 1611, that Johann Kepler first recognised that 'snow-flowers' had an essential unity of pattern in their symmetrical hexagonal form. In one of his books Needham points out that the Chinese contribution goes back to a tenth-century encyclopaedia entry, which preserves a passage in a book written by Han Ying from about 135 BC. Nothing much was made of this sound observation because six was the number associated with water: snow was 'the extreme form of Yin'. In Europe, on the other hand, the natural six-pointedness of snowflakes was not observed until the Renaissance, after which knowledge about it and many other phenomena rapidly increased. It is a wonderfully blown image upon which to tell the tangled history of a civilisation.

Needham's personal life was on the up too. Lu Gwei-djen was living close by again, just a few yards away from the house he shared with his wife, in an arrangement that suited all parties concerned. In 1959, he was elected to the presidency of the fellows at Caius, an almost unimaginable reversal of events earlier in the decade. Later to become master of the college, he proved to be a traditionalist while remaining perfectly left-liberal in his support for the Progressive League, the New Left Review Club and the Campaign for Nuclear Disarmament. But he was slow to criticise the Great Helmsman Mao, even though his correspondents and scholars generally were suffering greatly from the asperities of the Cultural Revolution.

Surrounded by a forest of documents, Needham was beginning

to realise that he might not manage to recreate ancient Chinese society in its entirety within his lifetime. Some of the seven volumes were calving fascicles. He brought in collaborators, and the work is still going strong: publication proceeds under the guidance of the Needham Research Institute (NRI), which has just released part 11 of volume V, on ferrous metallurgy. The NRI had been set up at Cambridge by the ailing sinologist in 1987, after years on the fund-raising circuit. His library had to be housed somewhere, after all. His ailing wife died that year too, fifteen years after publishing her own magnum opus *Machina Carnis*, an account of the biochemistry of muscular contraction. In September 1989, in a small ceremony at the college chapel, an ancient figure married the woman whose love had inspired him so many years before. Lu Gwei-djen, aged eighty-seven, was to die not long after, and Needham himself, now a Companion of Honour, died, as old as the century, in 1995.

Needham would hardly be surprised at the dynamic explosion of wealth and creativity in China, even in the decade or so since his death, since that creativity was implicit in his 'discovery' of China itself. He was chronicling a cultural self-confidence as well as a technological past that had been completely hidden—'the unique degree of self-knowledge that helps to make China *China*'. Winchester's biography fails to explain the shift in Needham's interests: there is less of a disruption than the reader might otherwise suppose between his achievements in chemical embryology and Chinese civilisation. The country to which he devoted the later part of his life allowed him to examine how levels of complexity, process and relation had come together in the past in something that resembled his projection of the future good society. Not all sinologists or historians agree with Needham's categories, which have their sources in Western thinking, nor with his diffusionist approach, which awards precedence to China on the basis of historiographic record and then sets out to affirm how the technology in question subsequently spread across the world. Diffusionism, with its belief in the essential unity of science, makes no allowance for the possibility that innovations may be punctual or parallel, occurring independently of the social faith we call progress, which Needham had in bags; they may even be lost, if only temporarily, to history. Besides, relying so heavily on historiography scants the achievements of other ancient civilisations, such as India's, which left fewer records.

It remains to be seen whether China, which has gone through so many dynastic cycles and been bureaucratic since its feudal beginnings, will absorb the twenty-first century into its own history or whether, in undergoing a sped-up version of the industrial revolution's war on Nature (it took Britain three-quarters of a century to increase its GDP fourfold, China has multiplied its GDP *ten*fold in only twenty-five years), it has abandoned its ancient cosmology and been engulfed by that troubling western hunger for the ends of things. A certain Captain Ahab heaves into view.

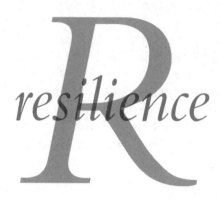

resilience

A Mining Town in Australia

THE WORKING LIFE AS A MATTER OF CONSCIENCE
AND FAITH

Broken Hill is a nondescript town in the far west of New South
Wales that lies over a thousand kilometres from Sydney, so distant
from the state capital that it prefers to keep South Australian time.
The typical postcard view of the city is an aerial one taken from
a Flying Doctor plane, where it looks like a tiny circuit board
stranded in an almost flat straggly-brown expanse of outback
stretching to the horizon; only when the plane begins to descend
towards the small local airport do you start to see furrows and
ridges, skeletal trees, the bleach of salt lakes and claypans, the odd
startled emu. In this vast dry bed west of the Darling River there
are only one or two signs of human habitation, the corrugated iron
roof of a farm or an out-station: Broken Hill lies out there in the
big red, and hugs its isolation. The town lacks the conventional
markers of the picturesque but its history and character are exemplary in a country that prides itself on the adaptability of its people.

I was a Medical Officer at Broken Hill Base Hospital for a year between 1990 and 1991, which meant being a kind of dogsbody; but there were few areas of medicine I didn't touch on in that year. I learned to treat problems of a variety and type I'd never met in textbooks. It was the kind of experience that left my heart in my mouth at times, other people's hearts often being in my hands, but relief at getting things right buoyed me through fatigue and worry. For several months I was duty officer in casualty by day, and up at night to learn from the midwives, and sometimes there were entire fortnights when I never got an uninterrupted night's sleep. Lack of staff forced those of us who were there to work long hours, which was irksome since I seldom had time to observe the country around me as much as I would have liked.

But I did notice a few things.

There were, all told, four directions to go from Broken Hill. Bush, which was anywhere in the four-wheeled zones that lay due north, west, and east; downriver, sheer poetic licence since the Darling river from which the town derived its drinking water ran at its closest point nearly a hundred kilometres to the east; and t'Adelaide, where the Flying Doctors would take you to the General Hospital for surgical repair if you sliced your tendons—those were the original three. Then there was the pervasive Broken Hill byname: *You from Away?*

Away was indeed my provenance. Away started a few hundred kilometres from Broken Hill, at Cobar on the Sydney road, hovered around the affluent Murray and Darling rivers on the Victoria border, extended a little into neighbouring South Australia, and meandered on rugged, men-only holidays fishing for the freshwater crustaceans called yabbies up along the dingo fence in Cooper's Creek, abutting Queensland. One of the world's most remote river systems, this collection of transient waterholes with its shelter of coolibah trees and lush vegetation had rescued the explorer Sturt from the relentless heat in 1845, on one of his attempts to find Australia's inland sea.

There was, of course, another—unstated—way to go. That was underground. It came too as a permanent option for some of the older miners, since gravity is a force so strong it eventually drags all living things under the earth's cuticle. 'In nations as in geology,' wrote the French historian Jules Michelet, 'warmth is down below. Descend, and you will find that it increases; in the lower levels, it is burning hot.'

I went underground once, just for a day, in the South Mines, down to level twenty-five. Level twenty-five was a kilometre under the surface of the earth. It was black, damp and very warm. 'I was obliged to do it', wrote the German writer Heinrich von Kleist in 1801 about going down the mines at Freiberg in Saxony, in what had become a rite of passage for German writers in the Romantic era, 'so that when I'm asked "have you been there?" I can answer: yes.' Like Kleist, I wanted to say 'yes', so I clad myself in gumboots to protect my feet and a hard-hat to take any knocks. A few weeks before, I'd read Fanny Kemble's diary entry on her visit to the excavations for the Thames Tunnel in 1827: she was nearly overcome by an 'indescribable feeling of subterranean vastness'. She, however, was about to enter the age of the technological sublime; here in the mechanised gloom, it was decidedly post-heroic.

What I could see was a smooth functioning warren of cables and sewers and service tunnels. Giant mastodons came up the ramp from below, their lights flaring. Most of the miners' work had been automated and seemed to be entirely given over to running and monitoring machines, rather than coming muscle to stone with the rockface. You would have to go back and read Orwell on the 'fillers', in 1937, to get an impression of the sheer physical dint involved in cutting out a mountain from the inside. The miners he describes had to crouch down on their knees and shovel for seven and half hours, with one short break for bread and dripping and a flask of cold tea. He talks about the oppressive heat too, and the fierce blasts of air let out by opening the fire doors, and the distances the men had to trudge underground. That was mining at the end of the second technological revolution, when humans still manipulated matter with their bare hands. Mining, like farming and building, is one of those forms of work in which the worker is himself significantly altered by what he does; his posture, gait and build are never the same again after he has 'worked' on the world.

But the machines weren't always predictable, nor was the seam. I'd had calls in the early morning at the hospital, when the emergency room waited for a crushed miner to be driven up from the several levels beneath ground; and there was the occasion when I'd had to wait at the mine-shaft for a thirty-year old to be winched up from the passage where he'd collapsed. He was blue where his skin could be seen through a film of dust, his eyes fixed and dilated and there was nothing I could do. His heart, that fish on a lead, had stopped jumping a good twenty minutes before.

The pensioners, the ones who stayed in the town when their money came through, and they weren't many, would talk about how things had been in the old days. Life had been pretty awful.

In the mid–1880s a boundary rider called Charles Rasp discovered the tip of a hangar of ore in the Barrier Range that would prove to be the world's largest seam of silver, lead and zinc: a few years later over nine thousand men working in ten mines were supplying ten percent of the world's lead and eight percent of its silver. The orebody was shaped like a coat-hanger, its neck the outcrop of 'broken hill' from which the town got its name. Rasp and the other outriders who became his partners lacked the expertise to make much of the discovery and the rights were sold to a group of pastoralists who founded the Broken Hill Proprietary Company. Edward Stokes, the town's gazetteer in his photographic record of the town in its hardest years, *United We Stand*, put the company's wealth at a conservative eight million pounds by the end of the decade. BHP's dividends established heavy industry in the country and were one of the major factors in making Australia the country with the highest living standard in the world in 1900: many Australians are unaware of this fact and those who are recall it with irony. And BHP is the country's one truly international company, though the name of the town is a ghost inside the acronym. But clearly minerals and fossil fuels were instrumental in transforming what were toe-hold colonies into modern nation-continents, and in this the opening of the Australian interior has much in common with the settlement of the American West.

The whole history of Broken Hill was one-way: lots of money out, and precious little in. Few of the mine proprietors had their residences built in the town. W. H. Patton, the BHP manager in 1899, refused to open the new hospital; it was characteristic of his disdain for this inhospitable place and the miners who worked the seam. After the 1909 lockout, BHP was regarded with sarcasm and bitter contempt in the town that had made it wealthy.

And the region was inhospitable. In summer the temperature was a constant 100 Fahrenheit and above. Rain was scanty; the nearest river a couple of days away. There was the torment of the bushfly, *musca vetustissima*: its passion for bodily orifices had been noted centuries before by William Dampier, one of the first Europeans to stumble across the continent. Everything had to be shipped up the road from Adelaide, over three hundred miles. In winter and spring the prevailing westerlies blew unimpeded across the scrub, which had been laid waste by almost complete deforest-ation and overgrazing, and whipped up huge billowing sandstorms that could be seen in their ominous approach an hour before they hit the town. The mobile rampart of sand blocked out the sun and choked the lungs, driving flocks of panicky birds any which way in the preternatural stillness that rides ahead of pandemonium. A storm mighty as a deity heaved great eddies of dust from the slags of lead and zinc tailings next to the mineshafts, and made men and women tremble for their lives. The earth was in the sky. Movables were battened down, the animals taken in, the windows sealed. And still the dust crept into the houses—through the ventilation slats, through minute cracks in the walls—and left a thick toxic rime on the tables and chairs.

I experienced a pipsqueak descendant of one of these sand-storms myself one cold July morning shortly after arriving: it was a nagging, tugging wind that barely lasted an hour and though it threatened at times to rip off the roof it was certainly nothing like as fearsome as the rolling dust storms that had entered collective memory, most famously in 1907 when the town's first professional photographer, within weeks of arriving, caught his first scoop: a menacing black nimbus of dirt rising up behind the Trades Hall. Nonetheless, this hour-long storm was rude enough to expose our house as the flimsy tin-walled construction it was; it brought to mind Lillian Gish struggling against the eight aeroplane propellers used to drum up the north wind in the famous pre-talkie film *The Wind*, in which she and her lover are a hopelessly fragile pair in the lulling core of the maelstrom. The visual power of the film, it was apparent to me when I saw it once on television, would have been swamped by sound-effects.

A different dust killed miners. The old train station in Sulphide Street had been converted into a museum and one room filled with old technology from the hospital. Iron lungs were displayed in every corner. These were required for the miners who developed pneumoconiosis and progressive fibrosis of the lungs because of the dry drilling. Safety measures were non-existent. Kerosene lamps lit the shaft landing areas but candles were the main source of illumination until about 1911, when carbide lamps were introduced. It is easy to imagine how intimately a miner would have to know his orebody, replacing sight with a keen sense of touch and vibration. 'You'd tap her, try the ground', confirms one old miner in Stokes' book, categorising anything in nature that was fickle or difficult to handle as female—I remember one of my patients, who'd taken off his index finger while doing some repair work on his fence, sexing the culprit chain-saw even as he gingerly unwound the improvised bandage from his mangled hand—'and the ground was groanin' and talkin''. Other fatalities were due to the regular cave-ins (blasts and mine fires were less common since, unlike coal deposits, the lode did not produce explosive gases); men ended up crushed beneath huge boulders and slabs of rock. Between 1906 and 1913 one hundred and forty-five men died in the mines. Without running water or sewerage, the families suffered too: typhoid epidemics regularly claimed scores of infant lives.

The population then stood at thirty thousand. Broken Hill became, through want of an alternative arrangement, a self-governing municipality. On paper it was part of New South Wales, but the State Government had little interest in such a remote outpost and the town made its own disdain of Sydney ostentatiously clear. The mayor Jabez Wright refused to attend the celebration of the federation of states into the Commonwealth of Australia in 1901. 'I have something more important to do than attend the National Drunk', read the message he sent by telegram. The resentment was long-standing: the state government had refused to build a railway to connect Broken Hill with the South Australian narrow-gauge system that ran to the border, scarcely thirty miles away; and it was only when a consortium called The Silverton Tramway Company built a connecting line in 1888 that the city was released from its isolation. By the turn of the century Broken Hill was a small town that had organised itself well beyond the cargo stage of human settlement described in Gabriel Márquez's *Leaf Storm*: 'Even the dregs of the cities' sad love come to us in the whirlwind and built small wooden houses where at first a corner and half-cot were a dismal home for the night, and then a noisy clandestine street, and then a whole inner village of tolerance within the town.'

Two newspapers were established, one of which—The Barrier Daily Truth—is still publishing. Houses with their corrugated tin roofs and thin walls were built along parched green avenues and gum trees. The town took on a grid form, and the streets were named after the chemicals associated with mining and extraction: Bromide (our street), Blende, Argent, Cobalt, Oxide, Chloride. The poet Auden, who prided himself on his knowledge of mining lore and mentioned Broken Hill in one of his early dramatic pieces of the 1930s, would have been delighted by the nomenclature. A brewery was set up; there was a Theatre Royal, a score of hotels, any number of watering holes, a brass band… it was the beginning of a hundred years of going it alone.

The inner village of tolerance, as far as it went, stopped at the city limits where the desert started. Beyond was the Commonwealth of Australia: the Municipality of the Hill stood with its crisscrossing streets and patches of sunlight and refused to look any farther than the rows of quondong trees and municipal parks planted in the south to act as a windbreak against the duststorms.

The difference between the Australia littoral—one of the most densely populated areas on Earth—and the interior, the bush, was so striking that I registered the difference and some of the resentments that exist between city and bush within a first few days of arriving in the country. There were people I met in Melbourne who'd never heard of, or didn't seem to want to hear about, Broken Hill: for many Australians, their continent still has a 'dead heart'. Some people in the Hill wouldn't give a Sydneysider the time of day. After a while, I started calling where we lived Quarantina; I speculated what a continental people like the French or Russians might have made of the Australian scrub if they had been its exploiters rather than the British. They might have called it Erytheia, land of red dirt. The inertia induced by a landscape that stretches on and on into the remote distance is surely a species of

Oblomovshchina—a word derived from the name of the lethargic main character in the famous novel by Goncharov. And the French dream of a glittering and bounteous Lake Chad in the middle of the Sahara that would feed the greedy boilers of the locomotives of the Trans-Saharan Railway bears ready comparison with the desperate search for Australia's inland sea. But would the Russians or French have reacted differently to the mining towns? I doubt it: it seems a safe generalisation that ours is a civilisation that doesn't want to know to whom it owes its graceful lifestyle. Who needs the red centre except for its minerals, a townie might shrug his shoulders; leave it to the reprobates, solitaries and misfits, so we can get on with the business of being liberal. At any account, it seemed as if contemporary Australians were still a long way from the feeling caught in its fright by C. E. W. Bean: 'The Australian comes in the end to the mysterious half-desert country [...] And the life of this mysterious country will affect the Australian imagination much as the life of the sea has affected the English.'

In the year of 1908–9 wages were docked to below the subsistence level. The company's response to a court order requiring it to pay a minimum wage was to shut down production for two years. The town became a police state during the First World War, when the miners refused the draft. At the end of the war, they went on strike for nineteen months. The concluding chapter of *United We Stand* tells the remarkable story of that period of resistance and final triumph. The hospital became a relief station. Women miscarried; children developed malnutrition and child mortality increased by fifty percent; rent ceased to be paid, and people lived on a diet of bread, margarine, onions and potatoes. Every day the band went out and marched down Argent Street with most of the townsfolk behind the Union's banner. Troops lined the streets, and there were running battles.

In the end the radical miners who had organised the Big Strike won, because no one else was prepared to do the work. The gum trees shed their bark along the Adelaide road and Bartley's Barrier Band polished their instruments and went out in the heat and blood got shed on the streets as well as underground; but the message had reached home. It was just as Kafka, writer and insurance claims evaluator, formulated it in his report 'Commune of Workers without Private Property' (1918)—'the working life as a matter of conscience and a matter of faith in one's fellow man'. No activity involving human lives is ever entirely undeserving of attention, even if Kafka's phrase represents the kind of seriousness that comes late to human structures. In one of Chekhov's stories an idealistic young man decides not to work in a government office, but instead to seek honour in manual labour. He gets a job tiling roofs and painting houses: 'I was living now among people to whom labour was obligatory [...] and who worked like cart-horses, often with no idea of the moral significance of labour, and indeed, never using the word "labour" in conversation at all.' He has taken on in an almost frivolous mood of acceptance what those who work all their lives shoulder involuntarily.

When the miners won, what they obtained were the most advanced working conditions anywhere in the industrial world. The working week was restricted to thirty-five hours. Giant ducts and air filters were built to extract the dust that killed so slowly and invidiously. The night shift was curtailed, since this was when most of the accidents happened. Explosives were fired at the end of each shift, and the men would wait for an hour until the debris had settled.

This created a closed shop well before the letter in Broken Hill. The Barrier Industrial Council—the Union's new name—became the de facto government of the town. It hired and blackballed men, set prices in the shops, published a newspaper, regulated gambling hours and determined when the bottle shops could open. Since none of the tycoons who had made a bonanza out of the town ever built a mansion in it, the 'Second Empire' building of the Trades Hall with its mansards and metal roof and stately palm-trees became the one building in the town that suggested wealth or permanence. The 'living wage' would be negotiated here every three years by the union delegates and the companies. That was the only item on the agenda subject to negotiation: the health and safety measures of 1920 were to stay, almost as the town's charter, and the Miners' Pneumoconiosis Society in Oxide Street preserves the statistics showing the dramatic fall in mortality among their members after the dust was properly evacuated.

All of which meant that Broken Hill was a relic in contemporary Australia: a shrine to mateship and restrictive work practices. Jobs were scarce when I was there, a slide which had started in the early eighties and showed no signs of slackening off. The hospital was the second biggest employer in the town, and the month after I left they made forty nurses redundant. The Industrial Council used to pay inducements to doctors to come to the Hill; all that had gone well before my time. About five thousand people were variously out of work or retrenched or on slack time. There was a lot of illness in the town: lobar pneumonia, poorly controlled diabetes, alcoholic heart disease, dysfunctional families. In 1986, the companies tried to reverse some of the working practices secured over half-a-century before; there were certainly men doing the night shift when I was there, and blasting went on while the men remained underground in the canteens.

Global economics had made mining some of the poorer seams of less financial interest for the companies; in other words, the yield wasn't high enough to justify the expense of hauling it out of the ground. So they started reworking the slagheaps, the biggest of which stood like a small table mountain behind the railway line from Sydney to Adelaide: the tailings from the old days still contained twelve or thirteen percent silver and zinc. This stirred up clouds of lead that settled on the town and created a generation of dogs with poor control of their hind legs, which didn't impress the RSPCA or the townspeople: Public health inspectors came and went, dismissing the risk of lead poisoning in the children unless they went down on all fours like the town dogs and starting licking the ground. It was a folk memory. One biblically-minded indefatigable old miner I knew actually called his dog Neb, short for Nebuchadnezzar—his father had made sure he would never forget the time, a hundred years before, when smelters in the town and dry-boring in the mines had made lead poisoning a real threat, and no cats or dogs were to be found at all in certain parts of town.

Isolation and fear of losing a job made tough men malleable. Up the road, past the cemetery on Rakow Road with its bleak scrub and rows of miners' graves, was the premonition that haunted Broken Hill: Silverton. Silverton had once been a mining town like Broken Hill; it had had a population of three thousand in 1885 and solid stone-fronted buildings, and then the mining companies had decided that the new town to the south-east was more interesting and that was the end of Silverton. Silverton was a ghost town; it had a pub with a few real locals and a spillover of tourists who came to see where they'd filmed *Mad Max II* and *Razor-back* and the Castlemaine XXXX advert with the lager-drinking parrot, though word in the pub was that it couldn't stand the stuff. It was where the Broken Hill people would go if they felt a need to commune with the bush but didn't want the inconvenience of packing their four-wheel drives for the weekend. A little promontory looked out over the Mundi Mundi plains; people would park their cars there just before sunset, sit on the bonnets with a bottle of beer, and stare out as far as they could across the flatness until the sun was a deep red afterglow and coolness came up off the rocks. Beyond the horizon, in the direction they were facing, was Mount Hopeless, so called by the explorer Edward Eyre in 1840 when a belt of salt lakes prevented him from venturing further towards the centre of the continent.

A hundred years later, it looked as if Broken Hill might go the same way as Silverton. After all, the capital of the 'Indies', one of the most famous cities in the world after the Spanish conquest of the Aztec and Inca empires, had disappeared into oblivion, along with its lode of silver, six miles across; it had been worked out by 1730. Situated high in the Andes in what would later become Bolivia, Potosí, with its garish wind furnaces and freezing rock pits was, according to its historians, hell on earth.

In the belly of the beast, I was now being driven in a shuttle up a long ramp with a solid cylindrical sheath of concrete and bundles of cables pinned at intervals to the wall. I looked at the shape they made with their machines, their bodies trembling as they drilled into and prised loose the orebody; the machines products of the same hard material they had to cut and blast, inimical to the human shapes dragging it out of time. These ores were the planet's memory. It seemed small-scale awesomeness, the height of the tunnel making the figures of the miners look odd, macro-cephalic, with their gumboots and overalls and steel cables coiled around their shoulders. It wasn't entirely dissimilar, I thought for a moment, to what I did in the hospital on Tuesdays and Fridays, when I assisted the surgeon, introducing an endoscope with its little fibreoptic bougie down into someone's intestine, a long snaking push through the oesophagus and into the vault-like sump of the stomach, a receptacle with its own groundwater and slurry.

I had to walk the rest of the way up the gob road to the stope—a huge cavernous working area. It was uncomfortably hot and the noise of machinery was constant. It seemed as if I was in the Paris catacombs restyled by Le Corbusier as a huge inverted skyscraper, and I had a sudden vision of the town on the surface pinned down to the surface like Gulliver. No one, looking at this unsteady town shimmering under the sky, would ever believe a kilometre-deep ballast prevented it from being traded to the desert like a mirage. Its layers were so ancient they went back to before life on Earth: there was nothing organic trapped within them, not a single fossil; and the only biomorphic beast around was a giant mechanical mollusc drilling into the seam in front, showering huge slabs of dark ore to the side. Usually the blasters lined the face with explosives and let them loosen the seam, before they prised it free; here they seemed to drilling a connecting passage between two levels. Had I wanted to ask I couldn't have, since there was no way of making myself heard.

The days when miners brought their sprawlers and poppers down like exclamation marks on a hard intractable substance were long gone. Here, though, was where the sense of political cohesion had developed that translated into solidarity above ground; in tunnels that collapsed, in bad air, in grime, in massed assault, in the vertical time of the revolution, inside 'Nature's womb'.

It was still an activity that compelled imaginative assent. But it needed an elastic imagination to see all the strata where they worked, rested and played cards and darts as the different layers of Salomon's House in Bacon's *New Atlantis*, the underground chambers of which were six hundred fathoms deep. 'These caves we call the lower region. And we use them for all coagulations, indurations, refrigerations, and conservations of bodies. We use them likewise for the imitation of natural mines and the producing also of new artificial metals, by compositions and materials which we use and lay there for many years.' Underground was dark and archaic. At ground level, there was the mounting heap of rejected awareness. After Victor Hugo's *Les Misérables*, the fictional journey into the depths of the earth also extended into society, with the vision of society perched on a vast, dispensable and poorly defined 'underclass' that was vindicated in H. G. Wells' subterranean anti-

Utopia *Things to Come*. Mining was where the intellectual met the tough, since before digging became a respectable intellectual pursuit—one of our command metaphors for knowledge itself—only marginals and slaves had to dig. There were no givens: in this job, reality was what the mind sought out and won for itself.

Giant life returned to size coming back up to the surface in an old lift used to carrying far heavier loads that wobbled as it came up. As if language itself had been under pressure underground, the small party of visitors all started speaking at once; it had been small-scale Jules Verne, but we had travelled down into the heart of the lode; one of the sources of Australia's wealth and a hidden city where the mind shucked off its own inertness.

On the surface the light was a shock, headachy and confusing. The South Mines enclosure looked bleached, our eyes recoiled. I felt a strange feeling of relief, as if I had doubted that I would return from the underground levels, and made a mental note to look up my Dante. 'Here sighs and lamentations resounded through the starless air, so that at first it made me weep. Strange tongues, horrible language, words of pain, tones of anger, voices loud and hoarse, and with these the sounds of hands, which made a tumult whirling through the air forever.'

Dostoevsky's man from a hole in the ground comes up to the light of the 'most abstract and intentional city in the world' spoiling for a fight, enticed by what the Nevsky Prospect holds out—freedom from the caste structure that keeps him at the bottom. He dares to think himself on a footing with his social better, the officer who has yet to register his existence (who walked through him, as Dostoevsky puts it). 'And lo and behold, the most astounding ideas dawned upon me! "What", I thought, "if I meet him and—don't move aside? What if I don't move aside on purpose, even if I were to bump into him? How would that be?" This audacious idea little by little took such a hold on me that it gave me no peace. I dreamt of it continually.' It's only when he risks his person, like the Broken Hill miners, and confronts the ruling class in the person of the officer that he steps into his dignity. Underground heroes are something like Proustian snobs, only stood on their heads.

I wondered how often the Broken Hill miners thought about what their grandfathers and grandmothers had risked to throw off the dead weight of the past and create the kind of ebullient Australia Australians take for granted. Broken Hill was the pivot of the country's modernity. Thinking themselves marginal would have been to adopt someone else's vantage point.

As for myself, I cherished that morning when I went down and came back up again. I was in search of something approachable and met a mountain. There are few thoughts closer to the borders of terror than imagining the effort of breathing with the weight of the earth's crust on top of you. When fear goes there's only shame and the packed atomic darkness that even Dostoevsky's underground man can't budge with his shoulder. I often think of those miners about to lose their jobs. They didn't think much of the work they did but they didn't know what they'd do without it. I liked their cragginess and I liked their wives. They couldn't understand what would drag anyone from 'away'—of their own free will—to this place on the edge of the world.

There was no lack of light in Broken Hill. Next day walking to work in blinding sunlight and flies, across a ground marred by dry salt, I thought of going underground as the mirror-activity to that of the man in Plato's cave who somehow wrenches free of the chain round his neck and goes out to contemplate the sun, only to go back in again to his comrades sitting observing the shadow-play in an icy Tartarus or Hades stuck like a tick on the rump of the earth. What he had seen was real. A mole-man, he lives strengthened by it, turning the light over and over in his mind till it becomes sheer flukish crystal. More than that. We set violence and reason over against each other. Plato tells us there is an affinity between them. Violence is the effort of the man chained in the cave to escape the dark and see the real.

Another writer who knew about mines and underground fires wrote that colours were light's sufferings, material the gods concealed themselves with. If so, minerals must be the earth's calluses, where it hauls itself over on its side—crystalline, nervy oxides propagated by attraction.

S

science (envy)

Lamplighters and Lucifactors

ON WRITING (ABOUT) SCIENCE

The world is a fluent place. Physicists borrow quarks from *Finnegans Wake* (itself an encyclopaedia of correspondences) and lend allusions of strangeness and flavour to particle behaviour; there are crashing computers and left-handed neutrinos, the selfish gene and parasitic DNA, the slaving principle in critical-point physics, and an efflorescence of colourfully violent Marvel comic imagery in cosmology; while, curiouser and curiouser still, in the very next room deconstructionists and comparative linguists adopt algebraic protocols, literary critics yield to indeterminacy and even social scientists acquire expertise in confidence intervals.

A mere thirty years ago this oddly engineered pangolin of spare-part imagery and transferred epithets would have been shot dead on hearsay, and its carcase quarantined by scare quotes. Nowadays anthropomorphic fiction-making has journalistic licence. In fact, the further we get from the year of Wittgenstein's death, 1951, the less inclined we seem to be to guard against it. 'The truth is much more serious than this fiction', he once remarked about the simple phrase 'the cussedness of things', needled (as it were) by the casual way human qualities get rubbed on to things. The implication, post-Wittgenstein, seems to be that fiction is as serious as truth, or that seriousness itself is a faulty qualifier of either truth or fiction.

Then again our society may be more adept than it knows at living with conflicting epistemologies: the history of technology is also a history of language, for the word technology itself, when first used in the time of Leibniz's *De Arte Combinatoria* and the universal language projects of Dalgarno and Wilkins, was a term applied uniquely to grammar—to the science of rhetoric. Three centuries later we are casually aware of how that formal syntactic manipulation of experience undermines the very need it determines: for the concrete. Walter Benjamin noticed this long before anyone else. In a letter to Gershom Scholem, he cited this passage from Eddington's *The Nature of the Physical World*: 'The plank has no solidity of substance. To step on it is like stepping on a swarm of flies. Shall I not slip through? No, if I venture to do so one of the flies hits me and gives me a boost up again; I fall again and am knocked upwards by another fly; and so on. I may hope that the net result will be that I remain about steady; but if unfortunately I should slip through the floor or be boosted too violently up to the ceiling, the occurrence would be, not a violation of the laws of Nature, but a rare coincidence...'. He goes on to make the telling connection: in all of literature he could find no passage quite so reminiscent of Kafka's prose. The old symbolic understandings have gone, the experimenter is a species of error in his own experiment.

This is the kind of unexpected correspondence that Professor Carey pounces on (although Eddington is represented here by an excerpt from his other writings), and one of the remote kinships that informs *The Faber Book of Science*. Science writing, for that is what a fussier title might have suggested—*The Faber Book of Popular Science* or *Story-Telling in Science* or *Literate Science*—has become a nearly fashionable genre; more and more writers are adopting scientific ideas, while more and more scientists find they can maintain a good income as popularising writers. The genre even has its house rag in the *Journal for the Public Understanding of Science*. While far from '[plotting] the development of modern science from Leonardo da Vinci to Chaos Theory' as the dust-jacket claims (what kind of book would that be?), Professor

Carey's anthology is both challenging and conciliatory. He isn't afraid to stick his neck out: '[science writers] have created a new kind of twentieth-century literature, which demands to be recognised as a separate genre, distinct from the old literary forms'.

What is this new genre? If it *is* separate then it has something to do with the specificity of what's being told. Scientists do the telling, and have to tell stories about science to people who are not scientists. While the goal of a general public understanding of science might have been still possible in the time of the *Edinburgh Review* and de Quincey (even then there were knockers), scientists least of all would presume such things possible now. Our ways of using words are too sectoral, too mutually exclusive. Scientists who write are guided by their readers' appetite for sensation and ignorance of the subject-matter: anything that emerges from such a process can only be second-rate art, and because the standards of scientific communication have ceased to bear any relation to what passes for good literature, cannot be very good science either. Texts that require a firm grasp of mathematics, like James Clerk Maxwell's brilliant work on the movement of gases and electromagnetism, resist glamorisation. Literature has no use for progress, and writers—who have no choice but to invent their own problems—cringe at the user-defined status enhancement packs scientists carry around on their backs like the academicians in Swift's Lagado (jargon). How can the paradigms of what Wittgenstein called 'our disgusting, soapy-water science' become the gorgeous bubbles of art? What can literature make of the impersonal? Is facticity a fetish worth having?

Between the obvious selections—Galileo on his telescope, Priestley on dephlogisticated air, Leuweenhoek on his little 'wolves', Ronald Ross' discovery of the malaria protozoon in the gastric tract of the Anopheles mosquito, Pierre and Marie Curie scouring pitchblende for radium in their backyard, the invention of electric light—the book contains well-edited extracts from Malthus and Erasmus Darwin, Huxley and Maxwell, a chillingly objective account of parasitic wasps immolating a cricket by Fabre (which Proust, closer to the source, uses waspishly himself in *Swann's Way*), Stephen Jay Gould's sad account of the doyen creationist Philip Gosse, Primo Levi's story of a carbon atom from *The Periodic Table*, Armstrong and Aldrin on their moon landing,

Oliver Sacks' classic case-history *The Man Who Mistook His Wife for a Hat*, and Richard Dawkins—'It is raining DNA outside.' We find science as knowledge, and science as method, and sometimes it's hard to tell the difference. Some very obscure journals have been ransacked for their booty. Kekulé's dream-inventions of the nature of enantiomers—handedness in chemistry—and the aromatic structure of benzene come from the *Journal of Chemical Education* 1958, 35: 211. (Kekulé's dream of the latter was to all intents a mythic reappearance of the alchemist's symbol Ouroboros, the snake swallowing its tail, and clearly too disreputable a source of enlightenment for the 1985 meeting of the American Chemical Association at which two participants flatly refused to accept his story, committed to print like the story of Newton's apple, long years after the event.) Max Born's article on quantum mechanics with its proleptically accurate machine-gun imagery is taken from his inaugural lecture at Edinburgh in 1936. Carey has discovered naturalistic impulses in odd places: Maeterlinck, Berlioz at the anatomy table, Steinbeck on sea cucumbers and lice, Orwell on toads, Calvino on a gecko's belly (but no Proust or Kafka on the airplane, and no Bouvard or Pécuchet, or Zola—the problem being, presumably, to know where to draw the line). Most satisfying of all, in many ways, are the editorial montages where Carey boxes unlikely characters into the framework of a common idea: Freud and Auden; Lamarck, Shaw and Richard Wilbur (it could have been Mandelstam); Lyell and Tennyson; and Roentgen's X-rays hauled up to apotheosis in the sanatorium on *The Magic Mountain*. We get lost, pleasantly enough, in detail.

To venture a first definition of this new genre, we would have to say that science writing bespeaks a kind of exceptionalism: it offers either exceptional individuals (Nobel-prize-winning sperm-donors) succumbing to the fairly standard temptation of the Promethean style ('The solution came to me in a flash', 'arrived out of the blue', 'hit me like a bomb'), or alternatively, humdrum scientists of modest literary talent in an exceptional situation (which hardly ever happens to be a laboratory). Above all, it has a problem distinguishing ends and means, since the goal of science under controlled conditions can rarely if ever have been to turn a phrase: the discipline of a science is quite a different order of experience from imaginative needs and wants.

A passage of Scientific Sublime of the second type entirely unknown to me comes from William Beebe's *Half Mile Down* (1934), an account of a record ocean-dive in a steel bathyscaphe, to depths previously thought lifeless:

> After a few minutes I sent up an order; and I knew that we were again sinking. The twilight (the word had become absurd, but I could coin no other) deepened, but we still spoke of its brilliance. It seemed to me that it must be like the last terrific upflare of a flame before it is quenched. I found we were both expecting at any moment to have it blown out, and to enter a zone of absolute darkness. But only by shutting my eyes and opening them again could I realize the terrible slowness of the change from dark blue to blacker blue. On the earth at night in moonlight I can always imagine the yellow of sunshine, the scarlet of invisible blossoms, but here, when the searchlight was off, yellow and orange and red were unthinkable. The blue which filled all space admitted no thought of other colors.

Beebe's passage is eerie and calm, a reconstruction after the event that has been worked on to render the shape of mythic time. Ideas become as heavy as objects, and objects lose their solidity. The literariness of the passage pulls the reader up short: what is striking about scientists generally is their naïve realism, their unselfconsciousness about the non-scientific implications of what they do. Something of the same reconstructive intensity happens in Nabokov's imagination, which rarely if ever functioned at normal atmospheric pressure. The stroke of a butterfly wing above the Oredezh river leads across the walls of time to the convolutes of the most pictorial of autobiographies, *Speak, Memory*, itself a 'diabolic' reworking of another memoir called *Conclusive Evidence*: 'by 1910, I had dreamed my way through the first volumes of Seitz's prodigious picture book *Die Gross-Schmetterlinge der Erde...*'

As a corollary to the boldness of predictive theory, overambition is almost the defining characteristic of modern literature. Much of twentieth-century literature is a running commentary of misunderstanding in the wake of the sciences. In some cases, the misunderstanding itself became the creative principle: William Carlos Williams developed his new American 'objectivism' on the assumption that conventional prosody was Newtonian and his freeing of the metrical fulcrum a shift not entirely dissimilar in its impact to Einsteinian relativity. More fool Williams, one might think, but Carey reproduces part of his very curious poem 'St Francis Einstein of the Daffodils' just to remind us that after Williams came an entire line of major misunderstanders: Zukofsky, Olson, Duncan and Creeley. Even though we may mock Williams' immodest assumption of relativity theory for his poetry, some of his poems *did* succeed in articulating a new appreciation of experience, with something like science's attitude to its material (take his wonderfully exact description of the cyclamen); and it's interesting to read Miroslav Holub's declaration—Holub being one of the very few who excel in both science and writing, and a countryman of Kafka to boot—that his first forays into poetry were made by applying the Williams maxim 'no ideas but in things'. As Holub might say, what poetry has come to be aware of is that it lacks any equivalent for the velocity of light.

One problem is that as science has expanded so has the guilt of literate people about their ignorance. W. H. Auden, who was an avid reader of precisely the type of Scientific American prose included in this book (if only, as someone once wickedly suggested, to see how things had moved on since Lucretius), practically admits that the humanist cupboard is bare: 'art is the spiritual life, made possible by science'. Nobody reads a novel nowadays to know how we live now, V. S. Naipaul once said (to Ronald Bryden): 'today, every man's experience of dislocation is so private that unless a writer absolutely matches that particular man's experience the writer seems very private and obscure'. Indeed, Carey suggests that ignorance of the natural world has become an aesthetic problem in the arts. He cites the blankness of his own honours students, all intelligent and articulate, but unable to tell him when discussing the speculative Donne line of 1612 (written sixteen years before the publication of Harvey's *De motu cordis*) how blood gets from one ventricle to the other. Comparing Richard Dawkins' *The Blind Watchmaker* entirely to its advantage with Martin Amis' *Einstein's Monsters* he states: 'from the point of view of late twentieth-century thought, Dawkins' book represents the instructed and Amis' the uninstructed imagination'. This is a moot point (and unfair on Amis; I would have rather he'd

rubbished Jeanette Winterson's pretentious *Written on the Body*),
and Haldane was saying much the same thing in the last great era
of scientific and literary exchange, before war snuffed it out.

Presumably there is more than one form of instructedness.
Wittgenstein once wrote: 'the popular science books written by
our scientists aren't the outcome of hard work, but are written
when they're resting on their laurels'. This is the Wittgenstein,
we should remember, who studied mechanical engineering at
Manchester, co-designed the house for his sister at 19 Kundman-
ngasse, and assassinated the old dream of a universal language.
He represents the view of science as an activity that stuns into
summation, or as Goethe put it in his argument with Newton,
'the empirico-mechanico-dogmatic torture chamber'.

There is little sense of the havoc this tradition of linguistic
scepticism once wreaked in the philosophy of science, perhaps
because Carey's scientists are predominantly Anglo-American. A
poet from the same culture as Wittgenstein, Hugo von Hofmann-
stahl, provided the most succinct statement of a man paralysed by
the failure of words to effect any kind of transaction with reality,
and it is no accident that young Lord Chandos should address his
fictional letter to Francis Bacon (who first invoked the authority of
nature against the tenets of scholasticism and is prominently placed
in Carey's foreword as an example of the instructed imagination).

Or take Robert Musil, one of two scientists to write a defining
novel of the twentieth century (the other is the Italian Carlo
Emilio Gadda). Two years after publishing his novel *Young Törless*
Musil completed his thesis on Ernst Mach's theories of causality
and scientific language. He never renounced his commitment
to a philosophically rigorous and scientifically informed way
of thinking. Realism was a way to gain reality for the novel in
competition with science, an aim itself derived from a bowdleri-
sation of the scientific paradigm; and while he upholds the intense
denominativeness typical of scientific discourse, his oeuvre deliberately abandons the unequivocality of a scientist's language, the
illusion it gives of always being in control. Even in Musil's time the
notion of science as disinterested activity was old hat. 'The truth
is', he has his protagonist Ulrich say, in that chapter in which it
dawns upon him that he is a man without qualities, 'that science
had developed a conception of hard, sober intellectual strength

that makes mankind's old metaphysical and moral notions simply unendurable, although all it can put in their place is the hope that a day, still distant, will come when a race of intellectual conquerors will descend into the valleys of spiritual fruitfulness.'

The problem science poses for modernity as Musil writes it, is not one of meaninglessness, but of valuelessness. The unfinished *The Man without Qualities* is an examination of the value of experience, and the metaphors by which its characters live. Even within his large novel the essay was always Musil's privileged mode. This is a problematic choice, since the essay as a mode sets out unaware exactly where it might end up, a reason for writing that is liable to have the person ostensibly holding the lead dragged away for what may be a very long digression indeed. 'What is truth; said jesting Pilate; and would not stay for an answer.' That was Francis Bacon, again, in the first great collection of essays in English. The essay is a didactic tease.

In light of which Carey could perhaps have included in his selection, as an example of humour in science, a wonderfully funny short parody by the French writer Georges Perec of the material-and-methods style of formal discourse scientists use when they talk to each other (Sir Peter Medawar bluntly called it 'calculated hypocrisy'), anonymous first-persons-plural addressing their dictaphones after a round of 'sacrifices' in the animal cages. 'Experimental demonstration of the tomatotopic organization in the Soprano (*Cantatrix sopranica L.*)' offers an analysis of throwing tomatoes at divas under controlled conditions, and can be found in the slim volume of the same name. Perec even had the courtesy to write it in that international vehicular language with the simple-Simon syntax known as English.

Tomatoes (*Tomato rungisia vulgaris*) were thrown by an automatic tomatothrower (Wait & See, 1972) monitored by an all-purpose laboratory computer (DID/92/85/P/331) operated on-line. Repetitive throwing allowed up to 9 projections per sec, thus mimicking the physiological conditions encountered by Sopranoes and other Singers on stage (Tebaldi, 1953). Care was taken to avoid missed projections on upper and/or lower limbs, trunk & buttocks. Only tomatoes affecting faces and necks were taken into account.

Control experiments were made with other projectiles, [such] as apple cores, cabbage runts, hats, roses, pumpkins, bullets, and ketchup (Heinz, 1952).

A kind of unintended humour, if not parody, is commonly found in science writing's major modes: the mind-stretching ('gee-whizz mode' corresponding to the traditional literary idea of the Sublime) or the explanatory ('faction'), which might, if we want to be fussy, be further subdivided into interpretative, resolutive or expository approaches. Since we have the Merton Professor of English acting as treasonous clerk, in Leavis' eyes at least, it would have been good to have known a little more about the formal structure of rhetoric in science (though in all fairness perhaps beyond the remit of the book), about the phoney feeling that creeps over many scientists when they are expected to discuss their discipline in non-specialist language. If the facts won't speak for themselves, then who or what does? What kind of a narrative is it that sets out to flatter the reader's ignorance? What happens to the peculiarly exacting literalism of scientists when they abandon the reality of phenomena? Don't we all live parallel to the age to science anyway?—although I know how aspirin works, I still haven't grasped what my neighbour up the road told me last week about cosmic microwave background radiation. It seems strangely appropriate that when asked to explain what he had just lectured on, the brilliant mathematician Paul Dirac repeated word for word the explanation he had given the first time.

Indeed, the sceptic might notice that any kind of science writing requiring more than a modicum of mathematics has long since been given up as a lost cause. Language is, of course, used metalinguistically in many sciences—as Stanislaw Lem, a glaring omission and one of the few writers who knew his way around axiology, might have said. The sceptical reader might also wonder at the many kinds of science explaining which sidestep language altogether. He might have tried explaining in words how the HIV virus specifically attaches to a cluster designation 4 (CD4) molecule on the surface of a T-lymphocte, or how 'chromosome walking' is initiated using an identified gene to pick out clones containing adjacent sequences; and having put the 'same' information in graphic form seen what a difference 'picture theory' makes to comprehension (Leonardo da Vinci had a related problem: he was an *uomo senza lettere* who couldn't communicate fully with the learned men of his time because he was unable to speak Latin). Our sceptic might be startled at the editor of this book cheerfully and willingly exposing himself to charges of first-order philosophical naiveté. He might feel much of current interest in science and writing is simply confused or misguided, and the conflation of genius and pop culture to be another Californianism. Hard science has to leave ambiguity and polysemy outside in the cloak-room; it requires semantically reliable words and sobriety, and any form of narrative which deliberately courts the metaphor, that tool of imitative magic, had better watch its step. If I remain faithful to a metaphor, wrote Kafka in the guise of his investigating dog pondering the mystery of his dogdom, 'then the goal of my aims, my questions, my enquiries, appears monstrous'. In another dimension: science writing easily becomes to science what Walt Disney is to fairy tales.

These kinds of arguments don't dismay Professor Carey. He does his best to make good those old taboos, anthropomorphism and animism, showing how the better science explainers use them adroitly to engage the reader's understanding. Instead of being embarrassed by animism, for example, he recruits it as an ally: we cannot help but invest our humanity in the things around us. Perhaps a more subtle Darwinian justification for the mixed genre approach to the language of science writing is the increasing recognition of how patterns emerge within non-equilibrium biological systems solely by virtue of the cooperative dynamics of the system itself; that the ordering parameters of culture and science might at a deep level work like those of language. Here our sceptic might add: and all myths reflect the societies they come from, including myths about language, and in the way they rank their ontological priorities reflect what a society refuses as much as what it accepts.

Science writing—like any kind of writing—is always risking the metaphor: it cannot help but be partially affected by the assumptions and imagery of its time, but then forgets that in a discussion about conflict in nature a metaphor—with its slippery, proximate, leap-frogging metapharand—is now being treated as a literal in human affairs.

Think of Copernicus and Kepler, or the severely rebuking

editor's note that Peacock inserted into his edition of Thomas Young's *Reply to the Animadversion of the Edinburgh Reviewers* of 1804 in which Young first developed the idea of the propagation of light as a waveform based on his experiments years earlier with sound in organ-pipes. The survival of the fittest in the struggle for life is also, as the *Encyclopedia britannica* entry reminds us, a metaphor: 'fittest' hardly ever implies a particulate genotype but an array of genotypes which enhance population survival; 'survival' does not require catastrophe to make for effective selection; and 'struggle' does not mean Achilles versus Hector. These are rhetorical terms; and in any case the entire expression chimes like a tautology. (Darwin actually argued for the comparative, the *fitter*, not the superlative: what may be beneficial under one set of circumstances may be a hindrance under another.) It is surely extraordinary too that 'selfish' has been used to characterise the gene, when what is intended is something like 'optimising'. No wonder the Tree of Life looks wormy. Fit metaphor is image *and* idea, as Aristotle said in his *Poetics*. At which level we might recognise Darwin's insight, *sub specie linguae*, to be the flip-side of Ovid's continuity of forms (and note in passing that metamorphosis was Kafka's way of *purifying* his writing of metaphor). It is a characteristic of pseudo-science that it relies on the suggestive force of words rather than hard instances or actual models.

There are disappointingly few poems in this anthology. Professor Carey claims there are very few poems 'about' science *tout court*: he should read more poetry. He includes a piece of dated bluster by Ted Hughes which illustrates all the worst anthropomorphic aspects of being awed by science, but inexplicably fails to include anything by Marianne Moore, A. R. Ammons, Amy Clampitt, Edwin Morgan, Holub himself ('Metaphors face extinction / in a situation which itself is a metaphor. / And the whales are facing extinction / in a situation which itself is a killer whale') or even James Fenton's campily ironic Victorian revampings of the Pitt-Rivers Museum and Lyell's *Principles of Geology* in his sequence *Exempla*. Francis Ponge's *Le parti pris de choses* is the closest thing the twentieth century offers to Lucretius, but it isn't here. Coleridge's quip is advanced as an explanation for poetry's bias against science: 'I believe the souls of 500 Sir Isaac Newtons would go to the making up of a Shakespeare or a Milton', and the lack of science-mindedness among poets attributed to an unjustified assumption of superiority. Yeats put it even more defiantly: 'The discoveries of science can never affect reality'; his reality, he meant. In fact, with the notable exception of Hugh MacDiarmid, most poets have avoided the heroic mode in science not because they feel superior to it, but exactly for the opposite reason, as Auden's humble-pie aphorism illustrates. There is a broad array of poems on science that would quite flatly gainsay both Coleridge and Yeats, proving that Wordsworth's famous prophecy in the preface to the 1800 *Lyrical Ballads* of the day when Science 'shall be ready to put on, as it were, a form of flesh and blood' has substance after all.

According to Professor Carey, science and theology are not mutually antagonistic since the latter 'might, without any paradox, be regarded as a science, committed to persistently questioning and reinterpreting the available evidence about God'. True enough; but the Bible does not present hypotheses, it affirms revealed truths. It was the church and science as *institutions* that were at loggerheads, for both were religion's claimants: what was the rationalistic essence of Protestantism became, a generation later, the Scientific Revolution. The most powerful impetus of the latter was the search for hidden divinity (as attested by every page of Newton or even Locke, with his Most Knowing Being), and even in the Enlightenment science was still entangled in the search for authority: pantheism made something of a comeback in the nineteenth century. Yet Musil noted that the human mind began to win its most tangible successes only when it jettisoned the notion of God. Even so, 'the notion that haunted him [The Man without Qualities] was this: "Suppose precisely this ungodliness were the appropriate contemporary way to God! Every age has its own way there, corresponding to its most potent spiritual resources: might it then not be our destiny, the destiny of an age of ingenious and enterprising experience, to reject all dreams, legends and sophistries solely because on the heights of discovery about the natural world we shall turn towards him again and shall begin to achieve a relationship based on experience?"' A recent broad survey suggested that about forty percent of American scientists believe in some kind of Supreme Being, exactly the same percentage as recorded in a similar survey at the start of the twentieth century.

On the other hand, Carey suggests science is an enterprise which, by its very mode of conviction, is fatally vulnerable to contamination by politics. Science's lack of place for moralizing—the very substance of politics—is, he asserts, a condition of its strength and purity. Who could doubt it? Even so, he blithely skirts any (Frankfurt School) idea that modern politics may have hatched out of the same disintegration of the social body as the technosciences, and ignores the troublesome complicity between violence and technology. Take, for example, the curious link between Pasteur's development of the germ theory and his hatred of mass society and socialism, which is mentioned in a brief biographical excerpt in the book. The scientific credentials of Pasteur's vindication of the germ theory were never at any point advanced or retarded by that hatred. But they were *deformed*; and half a century later we find Louis-Ferdinand Céline, doctor and novelist, risking the Pasteurian metaphor in one of his scabrous anti-semitic books where he talks about the Jews as a bacteriological inoculum. The recurrence of Pasteur's concept in such a debased, excessive form should suggest what is really at work. Myth in the modern scientific context tries to justify itself with facts, since facts always appears to mean something *by themselves*, thereby dispelling just those questions of value Musil was so interested in.

The implicit moral thrust to Carey's own argument is: we should be sparing with metaphor. Why add to the world's available reality when there's already so much there? The overinvestment in metaphor and magical technological energies characteristic of some science writing (some people call it science fiction, but it might just as profitably be called inverted archaeology) may simply be a way of hiding the essentially pedestrian nature of the original activity. I was gratified to find confirmation of this in Miroslav Holub's wonderfully breezy book *The Dimension of the Present Moment*, where he maintains that administrative duties, cleaning up, telephoning, waiting in queues and being a citizen effectively account for ninety-five percent of his working time, leaving a less than significant amount of time for interrogating the null hypothesis.

All things considered, there are some splendid texts in this book, none of them so preoccupied with discovery as to obliterate the hum of the real. Carey enlarges the imaginative boundaries of an issue that should be of pressing importance to our culture; there may simply not be enough unprejudiced participants. There is no better description of how we respond imaginatively to scientific explanations of our world than Lévi-Strauss' introduction to his book *Histoire de Lynx*: 'everything occurs as the converse of oral societies in which hard facts (*connaissances positives*) were very much inferior to the powers of the imagination. In our society, hard facts exceed the powers of the imagination to such an extent that the only resource of the imagination, incapable of apprehending the world even as it is being revealed to it, is to turn towards myth.' That is exactly what Musil expressed with aphoristic lucidity in *The Man Without Qualities*: 'we have gained in terms of reality and lost in terms of the dream'.

As things are, I prefer to read Kafka to Eddington, not necessarily because Eddington is a terrible old bore but because Kafka in his weightless way allows for what we might call the possibility of failure. That is the one quality in our long history of defamiliarisation with ourselves that science, and science writing all the more so, cannot risk. Science is a successfully unstable venture, successful *because* it is unstable. One crucial distinction between writing and science is that failure in the latter is kin, not just etymologically, to falsity. Where imaginative writing is helpless in the face of reality, it is only by trying and failing, and failing better, as Beckett tried to do again and again, that he encountered that sense of not-quite-arriving we call reality. The first writer to tell us that was another Irishman, Laurence Sterne, who, for all the literary high jinks he got up to as he journeyed around Europe in that age of lamplighters and lucifactors, kept insisting all we have is a 'terribly weak human voice'.

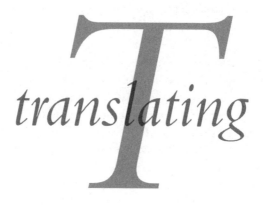

translating

Machine Made of Words

MEDICINE AND TRANSLATION

When I go through what I call euphemistically my archives, I find mounds of dog-eared A4, heat-sensitive fax paper and computer disks on subjects such as the following: fermentation techniques for monoclonal antibodies, nitric oxide (NO) as Molecule of the Year 1992, sterile loop ostomy bridges, French marketing chat about why pills that melt on the tongue are even more 'seductive' than pills that fizz in water, use of the Markov Model in cost-benefit analysis and heaps of CVs strewn with the historically-specific cultural insignia that really need an encyclopaedia to explain them, for example the French academic order 'Palmes académiques' or the German university title 'Privatdozent'.

That is a very small sample list of some subjects I've translated recently from my own source languages (SL), German and French, into English, the target language (TL) of about eighty-five percent of all biomedical translations. (A poet-friend of mine who also works as a translator insists on calling it 'host language', translation being for him more an act of faith or even a wager than a military directive.) The titles provide some idea of the multiple environments and disciplines that impinge on medicine and the biosciences: marketing, regulatory affairs, science journalism, production management, new products analysis—words that stare back in their strangeness. Often the human subject gets lost in this jungle of competing outlooks and deadlines; on the other hand, the titles suggest why translation can be a possible source of income, or even a profession: it freights the furniture of our time, technology.

Biomedical translation is a specialised form of translation, distinguishing itself from general translation by its reliance on terminology. Peter Newmark has estimated that specialist terms account for five to ten percent of a technical translation. That percentage will be much higher in a pharmacopoeia monograph than in a psychologist's report on the importance of restoring erectile function for psychic well-being in the average Frenchman. Out of necessity, since I often have to work in areas that skirt my basic field of competence, I keep and continually update glossaries of French and German words I encounter only rarely. In my experience the various Euroglot dictionaries on offer are not much use, being full of dodgy 'equivalents'—it might be 'physiopathologie' in French but it has to be 'pathophysiology' in English.

Many areas of human endeavour and interest have a rightful claim on technology, and even a grammar of objects supposedly stripped of emotive terms, sound-effects and metaphor still gets pulled every which way. George Orwell put it rather nicely: 'above the level of a railway guide, no text is ever quite free from aesthetic considerations'. I remember once being put out at having to translate a brochure for a German pharmaceutical company which carried the motto 'Let's join hands under these flowers against disease in this world': not only was the flower-image purple but it was also difficult to imagine a daisy chain of people being able to do much against that other chain: of cause and effect. French sometimes yields to the *poncif*—a kind of linguistic affectation that compels even technocrats, through fear of appearing ignorant of the real tradition, i.e. Ciceronian and humanist, to use archaic terms where something functional or declarative would have done just as well. Since few French scientists know Sanskrit, and since looking backwards is what distinguishes humanists from scientists, Greek is the highest god (or at least a kind of Aunt Sally). Hence such wonders of neologistic impulse as 'nycthémère' (twenty-four-hour period) or those intellectualising but mentally lazy suffixes ('-ismes').

A glance at my own files brings to light such curios as '*amyélé*' (pithed), '*lésion achromatique*' (non-staining gap), '*blutig bestimmen*' (measure by invasive method) and '*Haltungsanormalitäten*' (lack of motor coordination). Some of these terms are ordinary words co-opted to other denotative ends, others concept-terms or phrases that require formulaic repackaging. '*Chez la femme en période d'activité génitale*' ends up on a pack leaflet as the less fearsome 'in women of child-bearing age', which isn't quite the same thing, but is more revealing in the context (teratogenic effects of a drug on the foetus). Translators should never be afraid to omit empty phrases when translating. Concision is not the same thing as precision, but it can tighten a sloppy expression. Many orotund phrases in French are redundant and can be rendered with simple English prepositions, for example 'about' ('*de l'ordre de*') or 'in' ('*dans le cadre de*'); true to its clerkish soul, German has convoluted adjectival constructions that go on for ages by the simple trick of turning a participle into an adjective (see Mark Twain's essay 'The Awful German Language').

A dualist approach is often adopted when thinking about translation. Poetry translation approaches untranslatability; scientific translation hunts for the right Lego piece. One posits silence as the only thing mankind really holds in common; the other overrides philosophical niceties, since the results seem to work. For the technical translator, the act of translation is an exercise in impersonality and secular reality (a job for money)—rendering connotations, 'transcoding' professional or technical terms and improving the semantic clarity of the text, where necessary or possible. He is as free as any other translator to recast syntax, house-style permitting. He may often be more interested in getting the job done than in following the original, although in my experience it is impossible to work without first understanding both SL text and context. That would appear axiomatic, but I have sometimes been asked to salvage translations where it has been clear that the original translator didn't have the faintest notion of the subject matter. Part of the translator's ethics of competence includes knowing when *not* to translate.

Divergence and convergence are powerful forces that may be at work simultaneously within a language. English and French have been converging for the last century or so, and while German is remarkably hospitable to all kinds of specialist jargon from English, French often manages its own jargon: the acronym for Aids in French is Sida ('*syndrome d'immuno-déficience acquise*'). That a clinical term can be more and less than it seems—more stigmatising, less innocent—is instanced by 'sidaïque' (the adjective describing someone affected by Sida) which, rhyming with 'judaïque' ('Jewish'), was often heard on the lips of Le Pen and other French extreme right-wingers in the 1980s. Rather than risk that kind of infection, German phagocytoses most English acronyms, although others win through: nuclear magnetic resonance imaging (MRI) is 'Kernspintomographie', where the notion of 'Kernspin' is visually more dynamic and aurally more catchy in German than nuclear resonance, i.e. it makes an irresistible appeal to the *imagination*. The French for 'evidence-based medicine' entered the language in 1994 as 'médecine factuelle', which makes you wonder what was being practised beforehand.

What this suggests for the Euroglot translator is that the continent's languages are cognitively too close, although this closeness may be one reason why Esperanto survives as the only artificial language with a mass following, its substantives being almost but not quite familiar to anyone with a glancing philological interest in the history of European languages. It is not entirely irrelevant that Zamenhof, its Polish founder, was an ophthalmologist. On original publication in 1887 of his language project, Lingvo Internacia, he used the pseudonym Doktoro Esperanto (One Who Hopes); it was in fact this catchy pseudonym that took over as name for the language, an eponymic displacement phenomenon well known to the professional translator. The linguist Benjamin Lee Whorf called this cognitive proximity of the Romance and Germanic languages Standard Average European, and it is the ghost behind the very idea of translation in Europe: that it comes down to a process of lexical swapping, with a few minor syntactic modifications. Meaning is something that can be uncoupled and reassembled over and over again in a new linguistic form—'les découpes du même reel'. Accepting that languages are isomorphs reinforces a semantic fallacy that goes back to Aristotle: words are vocal tags attached by convention to things in a world supplied by Nature and identically conceptualised by the human mind. A meaning can then be lifted from its context and bodied in a different form because these different incarnations are rationally connected. It's as if we're all really thinking the same thoughts after all. But any person who has stepped out of his own language knows there are things he has to leave behind: if that weren't the case translators wouldn't have to struggle with the strictures of natural languages.

The Aristotelian view is omnipresent, however. It underpins machine translation (MT), or machine-assisted translation (MAT), the automated process of translating from one natural language to another. In the episode of the Grand Academy at Lagado in *Gulliver's Travels* Jonathan Swift was able to satirise the notion of a machine that could handle language. Three centuries later, after Orwell and on the whole rather less confident about the status of language as a uniquely human attribute—or rather, condemned to follow the logic of the metaphors about language we have engendered—we still rely on Turing's test as the best way to 'out' a machine: by getting it to answer a series of human questions. I once performed such a test on a MT programme and it spat out the term 'forward bedroom of the eye' for the French 'chambre antérieure de l'oeil' ('anterior chamber' in English too). I know of companies which use MT software to produce roughly usable versions of texts from Japanese or other distant languages, but for little else. On the other hand, the fact that we ourselves make increasingly little distinction between vital processes and techno-logical events (computer viruses and worms) might suggest to the uncritically conscious that the machines will soon be 'outing' the liveware.

Other factors impinge on the translator's autonomy. The power of transnational bodies like the EU has an increasing effect on *permissible* terminology. Although the term 'product licence' used to be a perfectly acceptable term for the statutory paperwork required by a medicine before it came on the market, Eurospeak dictates use of the unwieldy 'marketing authorisation' (by deri-vation from the French 'autorisation de mise sur la marché'); a drug itself is called a 'medicinal product'. Nothing, to an English-speaker, is quite so presumptuous as the official publication of the French state, *les Journées Officielles*, which prints sanctioned versions of new scientific terms; it is interesting to consult these publications with ten or twenty years' dust on them and note which words have had staying power. 'Endoprothèse' might be the sanctioned term for a 'stent' in French, a metal lattice device inserted via a catheter and expanded by the cardiac surgeon in order to keep a narrowed blood vessel open, but you'll be lucky to find it outside this essay.

English is a handy language for objects to come to voice in. Its furniture is more mobile than that of its other European languages. It is almost desexed. Scientific English prefers simple or co-ordinate to complex sentences, and even here some claim to detect the influence of the King James Bible (Hebrew part). It doesn't frown on, indeed may actively favour terms like *boil-off*, *shelf life*, *break-point*, *fit*, *doped* and *spiked* where more conventional latinisms are also available. I recently discovered *hot-melt* for thermoplastic and *step-down* for decremental in an American text. Geologists speak of *downbuckling* for subsiding and computer technicians use the term *handshake* for confirmation of a connection: the graphic quality of the term is a kind of non-verbal mnemonic—or *trigger*. Lakoff and Johnson point out that no natural language is exempt from buried intentionality: even in technical translations, you can find your-self running up against—a sporting phrasal verb itself!—the weird prominence of cricket and golf as imagistic sources for metaphoric terms in English.

But to be fair (the idea of *fair play* has hitched its way into all the European languages), and since I love both my source languages, I would point out that French and German have their own qualities. French neologises effortlessly—'morbimortalité', 'cathodique' (by analogy with 'catholique'), and the homophonic 'cédérom' are three recent examples—and German is adept at making sense with prepositions: take the basic root-term 'Blick' and add *aus-*, *ein-*, *durch-* or *über-*, or other substantives such as *Licht-* and *Augen-*, and six subtly related new words come into being. Here we have a source of that system-building other literary cultures find pedantic: the literary critic Walter Benjamin once observed that 'Mut' (courage) was a polarised word, being divided into 'Untermut' (stealth or cunning) and 'Übermut' (high spirits)—he was writing about fairy tales. German has the ability to project the brooding gestalt shape of its words so forcefully that their visceral meaning is 'understood' preverbally before a commensurate term can be found in the dictionary, or indeed in the mother-tongue.

I've also come to the conclusion, after several years in Europe, that the prepositions are the truly tricky parts of a standard European sentence. 'I'm interested in...' says the English speaker, while the French speaker 's'interesse de...' and the German 'interessiert sich für...' Prepositions are angels and pimps, the bits of language that get it going. J. S. Mill once observed that 'a large portion of all that perplexes and confuses metaphysical thought comes from a vague use of those small words'. Michel Serres, the maverick French philosopher of science, has written interestingly about our concentration on the heavy, substantive, material nature of the world to the detriment of the prepositional ability to give direction, mobility and relation. Prepositions trace relations rather than fix their position and contour. Serres' concentration on messages is, to say the least, intriguing given that knowledge in the sciences seems to be such a formidable cluster of substantives. Someone else once remarked that logical particles *and*, *or* and *but*—less noticed even than the prepositions—are the really subversive parts of language, an assertion that certainly bears thinking about. And Carlo Emilio Gadda, the Italian engineer-author, once complained that pronouns are the 'lice of thought' (*pidocchi del pensiero*), the filthiest of them all being the first person singular. Technical documents, with their inveterate habit of effacing personhood and avoiding the active voice, would seem to back him up.

While translating keeps a translator, by proxy, on the cutting edge of what's new—state of the art, so to speak—there are times when I feel like the American poet John Ashbery, who wrote a poem called 'The Instruction Manual' about a man translating a very boring technical file. The translator looks up to find his imagination running off to South America merely on the exotic sound of a city's name—'Guadalajara! City of rose-colored flowers!' But he conscientiously returns from his reverie to his instruction manual; and I can only suppose that doctors who end up in applied linguistics do a valuable job, since the practical application and extension of the sciences into Technology and Big Business require self-effacing types prepared to don the translator's traditional mantle of invisibility. But there's the rub: if a translator does his job properly, nobody notices; if not, then he has to put up with, at the very least, accusations of sleeping with the enemy.

Medicine itself can never get away from symbolic language, or abandon its lay orientation, and it is perhaps as well that most doctors are instinctively more attuned to the curse of babble than to knowing just where Broca's area is. Should you have another language and the time to apply it, working as a medical translator makes you even more acutely aware of how opaque the medium is. On the other hand, many doctors are unwittingly translators and interpreters anyway. Next time you have a quiet moment, read someone's medical history: it's nothing other than a formally explicit TL rendition of what for a patient may well have been a barely recountable SL script of threateningly inchoate bodily sensations.

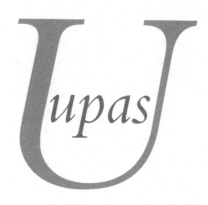

The Poison Tree

A JAVANESE BOTANICAL SHADOW–PLAY

The civic tree that would not grow

When I was studying medicine at the University of Glasgow, I came across an arresting title in the university bookshop that made me pick up the book for a second look. *The Upas Tree: Glasgow, 1875–1975* was a short history of the city written by the university's former professor of economic history and published by its press: indeed Sidney Checkland had probably taught my mother when she studied economics there in the 1950s. In the spectacular nineteenth-century growth of the hundreds of malodorous, blackened and often squalid tenements ('closes') that would house the workers who put their labour and lives into the industrial achievements of heavy engineering and shipbuilding—with Glasgow serving as 'a Liverpool and a Manchester together' long before the Clyde became a by-word for British engine power—and the ensuing slow painful twentieth-century contraction of the 'second city of the empire' due to its overreliance on a very specific set of floating capital, skills and goods and a corresponding failure to diversify, Checkland saw a paradigm for the decline of the United Kingdom as a whole, a process that had become seemingly unstoppable by 1981, the year of the book's second edition.

For all that his was a book centred on economic history, Checkland had chosen a symbol of natural growth to represent the city itself. The tree as a metaphor for human well-being—indeed as the fund of life itself—is a reassuringly solid one. Though humans are ambiguous creatures suspended between nature and culture, trees and their root systems are entrenched in our metaphors for being at home in the world. Buddha received enlightenment under a sacred fig or Bodhi tree, with its heart-shaped leaves. In Hinduism, the banyan tree is the resting place of the god Krishna—'and the Vedic hymns are its leaves'. Plato liked to discourse beneath the silver spears of an olive tree. Some Biblical commentators had Christ crucified on a tree, though they don't say which. Norse mythology had its famous warden tree, Yggdrasil. Even Jeremy Bentham had his 'tree of utility'.

But what was the *upas* tree?

The Shorter OED describes the upas tree as 'a fabulous Javanese tree so poisonous as to destroy life for many miles around'. It is a symbol that stands for anything exerting a baleful, destructive influence. Checkland was using the upas tree as a figure for the doldrums of the once proud shipbuilding and marine engineering capital of the world: Glasgow's determination to maintain its reputation for heavy engineering had come at the expense of everything else that ought to be 'growing' in the city. It was a particularly rich irony, since the coat of arms of the city bore a famous miracle tree that 'never grew', in the rhyme learned by generations of the city's schoolchildren, including myself. 'Now the Upas tree,' wrote Checkland, 'so long ailing, was itself decaying, its limbs falling away one by one. Not only had its growth been inimical to other growths, it had, by an inversion of its condition before 1914, brought about a limitation of its own performance.' By the mid-twentieth century, the city had become a byword for militancy and defensiveness. Like a piece of machinery itself, Glasgow had, in the words of Samuel Taylor Coleridge's famous expression, become a giant with one idea.

There was another sense in which the upas tree was a potent symbol of what industrial development had cost a city which, a hundred years before its modern expansion, had been declared by Daniel Defoe to be 'the cleanest and beautifullest' in the kingdom: the chemical industries set up in the 1820s around the Shawfield Works on Glasgow's southern approaches were to turn its water-meadows into the first industrial wastelands. The employees of this factory, which was established by John and James White on a twenty-acre site on the Rutherglen Road and was only one of the city's several huge chemical factories and iron foundries, were known as 'White's canaries' or 'White's dead men', depending on whether they had been working with sulphur or soda ash. 'There were the chrome furnacemen, the pearl ashmen, the crystal house men, the workers at the vitriol tanks, and the acid towers, together with the general labourers', writes Allan Massie in his short history of the city. 'The chemicals industry, indeed, in spite of being science-based, produced the nadir of working conditions, a scene of terrible male degradation.' Contemporary critics wrote about the dismal light and poor air, and the strange, bitter, blighting wind: Charles Dickens caught the atmosphere of all such places with his description of Coketown in *Hard Times*—the foul-smelling black canals, the serpents of smoke from tall chimneys, the pistons of the steam-engines working monotonously 'like the head of an elephant in a state of melancholy madness'. Industrial-ised or de-industrialised, there are devastated parts of the country, and not just the suburbs of Glasgow, that offer a 'Scotland so real it defies the imagination', in the words of the novelist James Robertson in *And the Land Lay Still*.

These were the strange fruits of that same science Coleridge had told his friend Humphry Davy in a letter of 1800 was the supremely human activity—and 'being necessarily performed with the passion of Hope, it was poetical'.

The exotic tree of permanent shadow
I hadn't spared a thought for the upas tree in twenty years when, in a dingy little second-hand bookshop at the side of a garish shopping complex on the Jalan Rasuna Saïd in 2005, the year of my first visit as a health consultant to Java's capital, Jakarta, a

city so large that its current population is at least ten times that of Glasgow at its peak of just over one million (but nobody is counting), I discovered a copy of a book called *The Poison Tree*. It was a translation of selected writings on the natural history of the Dutch East Indies (when Jakarta was known as Batavia) including a description of the upas tree, which had given the book its title, by an obscure naturalist with a curious name: Rumphius.

Rumphius was the Latinised name of a German naturalist from Hanau, Georg Eberhard Rumpf (1628–1702), who settled in the capital of the volcanic Banda Islands in the Moluccas (present-day Maluku), then the heart of Dutch trading operations in the archipelago. Rumphius worked for 'The Company', the metonym universally used to describe the formidable Dutch East Indies Company (VOC): he enlisted in its ranks as a gentleman soldier, leaving Europe in 1652. He would spend the rest of his life in Ambon (Amboyna), the main entrepot town in the Spice Islands from which the Dutch conducted and controlled their lucrative monopoly in cloves, pepper and nutmeg, which could sell in Europe for up to three hundred times the local purchase price. The first Europeans to moralise about materialism, the Dutch were ruthless in the defence of their economic interests on the Spice Islands, as the Portuguese and British and many rebellious Bandanese were to discover. Rumphius rose through the ranks, becoming a civil servant and establishing a reputation for himself as a man of ability and probity. He had talents as an architect, geometrician and linguist, but by the 1660s was known as a botanist and naturalist—a man who loved to devote himself to his 'curious studies'. By a cruel irony, even as he acquired a 'small parcel of land' near Fort Victoria on Ambon and the leisure he needed for his studies, he lost his sight, probably as a complication of glaucoma. For the remaining thirty years of his life he had to rely on 'borrowed eye and pen'. It didn't stop him dictating to his son and various secretaries some astonishingly delicate descriptions of the world around him; and some of these entries had been translated with brio, in the book I was holding, by the scholar E.M. Beekman.

Understandably, in view of his geographic remoteness from anything like a printing house, only one of Rumphius' writings was published in his lifetime, his account of the earthquake that killed his native wife and daughter in 1674. He gave his wife's name to an orchid with white lanceolate floral bracts they had found together: 'I call it *Flos Susannae* in Latin [...] in memory of her who when alive, was my first Companion and Helpmate in looking for herbs and plants': the Susanna Flower is now listed in the nomenclature as *Pecteilis susannae*. In all his work, Rumphius, like a twentieth-century ethnographer, always sought out sources of practical knowledge at the local level: he quizzed the *dukun* (the local healers), most of whom were women, on how they used plants, and ignored Galenic precepts entirely. And the women must have trusted him, because he writes about plants that were used for intimate hygiene or as abortifacients—women's secrets. Rumphius also wrote a history of Ambon, as well as reports on the island's agriculture, a lexicon of the Malay language (up to the letter P) and the several folios that constitute his *d'Amboinsche Rariteit-kamer*—his 'Ambonese Curiosity Cabinet'.

These were mere by-works in relation to his magnum opus, *The Ambonese Herbal*, the seven hundred chapters of which he finished in 1687. It is one of the great works of pre-Linnean naturalism. Beekman, a Dutchman who was a professor of Germanic languages at the University of Massachusetts, spent the latter part of his life translating all the significant works of Rumphius' considerable oeuvre. In his introduction to *The Poison Tree* he writes that he set out to use only words that were current before 1700, and in order to verify usage had to turn to the Quaker historian William Sewel's *A Large Dictionary of English-Dutch*, a book first published in Amsterdam in 1691. What has been lost to science has been reclaimed as literature, for Rumphius' personality is stamped all over his writing: his is a richly embodied language that preserves the individuality of everything he comes across. Osip Mandelstam's description of the experience of reading Linnaeus' *Systema Natura* conveys rather well the prose style of Rumphius' work, which Linnaeus (who concealed his sources) had probably read during his time in the Netherlands: 'It is Adam handing out certificates of merit to the mammals, having invoked the aid of a wizard from Baghdad and a Chinese monk.'

Rumphius' fabulous botany (which already relies on the economical use of binomials) is a reminder that one of the most powerful forces behind what is now called 'enlightenment' was the need to find an exact nomenclature and descriptive method for naming specimens from botany in particular and the natural world in general. Botany played a central role, as the substantial part of *materia medica* and an item of cultural baggage which had to be acquired by every educated person, in the development of modernity, bringing together medicine and science, commerce and expanding empire, and connecting them all with the new cognitive scope accorded to the eye by magnification and microscopy.

Evocation is one thing, systematic description another; Rumphius had a talent for both. Beekman's copious notes on what is a relatively obscure chapter of natural history make it doubly a pleasure to linger over Rumphius in translation: his translator is a knowledgeable guide not only to the natural phenomena and obscure customs of the Malay Archipelago but also to changing usage in English, German, Dutch, Malay and Chinese. If George Steiner could spot a resemblance between Joseph Needham's famous synoptic work *Science and Civilisation in China* and Marcel Proust's *A la Recherche du Temps Perdu* as documents of a civilisation grasped in the round, then there is a case to be made for Beekman's recreations of Rumphius' primordial epiphanies.

After a brief description of the 'spatter-poison', the bloody sap of the tree collected using bamboo conduits and smeared on arrow-tips for hunting game (and killing Dutch mercenaries), Rumphius writes: 'Under this tree and for a stone's throw around it, there grows neither grass nor leaves, nor any other trees, and the soil stays barren there, russet, and as if scorched.' The upas tree casts a dense meteorological shadow: it has a sinister climate all of its own. Birds unfortunate enough to alight on it can be found dead beneath it. All animals shun it except for a 'cackle-snake' that sometimes terrorises nearby villages, a kind of basilisk able to immobilise victims by gazing at them before destroying them with its mephitic breath.

What Rumphius was describing was the cryptobotany of the bark cloth tree, '*ancar*' in Malay or *Antiaris toxicaria* in botanical nomenclature, around which has grown, as Beekman comments, a 'tanglewood of lore and legend [...] most of it preposterous though marvellous as fiction'. A surgeon working for the Dutch East Indies Company in Semarang, N.P. Foersch, published in the *London Magazine* of December 1783 one of the first widely read accounts of the upas tree, embellishing his paper with several fantastic folk-tales about the terrible 'bohun upas' but providing no details about its botanical nature or even how the poison was prepared. It now seems that Foersch was a fictitious person and the letter itself a hoax perpetrated by the Shakespeare specialist and friend of Dr Johnson George Steevens, who was pandering to the eighteenth-century fascination with exotic tales; at any rate it was a literary mystification that gripped the Romantic imagination. The upas tree does indeed produce a toxic latex containing a cardiac glycoside that can cause a fatal arrhythmia, but its shade has never blasted the living in the manner either Rumphius or Foersch suggest: indeed it is considerably less malign than the West Indian manchineel (*Hippomane mancinella*), commonly found as a windbreak near coastal plains and beaches: its fruit and sap are among the most toxic on the planet.

It is the upas tree, though, which has entered myth.

The sentinel tree of the Arctic Circle

The malefic upas tree bewitched the poets of the early Romantic period, where the fascination may have been fed by references to it in Erasmus Darwin's poem 'The Botanic Garden', where it was called 'the *Hydra-tree* of death'. Coleridge wrote, 'It is a poison-tree, that pierced to the inmost, / Weeps only tears of poison.' The Victoria and Albert Museum in south London has a large, claustrophobic canvas titled *The Upas, or Poison Tree in the Island of Java*, based on Darwin's poem by the Irish artist Francis Danby, which was the sensation of the British Institution exhibition of 1820, only a few years after Stamford Raffles had been Lieutenant Governor of the island during the Napoleonic Wars and penned a dismissive note about Foersch's 'extravagant forgery' in his ency-clopaedic *The History of Java* (1817). Byron in 'Childe Harold's Pilgrimage' associated the tree with the 'uneradicable taint of sin'; Balzac, Southey, Charlotte Brontë, Dickens, Melville and Ruskin all had upas trees in their literary gardens. Even Blake imagined, in a pre-Freudian parable on the dangers of repression, an unspecified 'poison tree' growing in the garden of his mind: it had grown out of anger and its apples were likely to be toxic. Nothing could grow in its shade. The tree that brings death and not life leans out of the Romantic era and into the twentieth century as a self-poisoning of the mind: Friedrich Nietzsche would have recognised it, having in spite of his better intentions contributed to its upkeep, as the tree of resentment.

In fact, it was the celebrated Russian poet Alexander Pushkin, who in his somnambulistic poem 'Anchar', wrote the finest lyric on the upas tree—'The fearsome sentinel / Stands alone in all the world.' Only a black whirlwind dares to disturb the poison tree and it, in its turn, becomes pestilential. Where does the contagion stop? Even language itself, we suspect, might become the infectious vector of this primal curse. And sure enough, a man of power (Pushkin identifies him only as the Prince) sends another man ('a poor slave') by 'commanding glance' to gather the glassy coagulated resin that hardens in the night. The Prince has this gum spread on arrows and looses 'perdition through the air' on neighbours without access to an antidote, and who are in any case unacquainted with such ruthless methods of territorial acquisition.

Pushkin neglected to submit this poem to the censor for approval before its first publication in 1832 and consequently had dealings with Count Alexander von Benkendorff, director of Nicholas I's Third Section (internal police), now remembered if at all for his bizarre inability to remember his own name: he was alert enough however to notice that Pushkin had been bold enough to name outright the tyrant in the first version of the poem 'Tsar', the man to whom the history of the nation belongs. Not that anybody in Russia would have had any problems recognising who was meant in subsequent versions by 'the Prince'. In a critical study of Pushkin John Bayley wrote that, 'Anchar condenses its apprehension of power in a few heavy drops'—indeed, both the Prince and the tree are the grim guards of their redoubtable isolation. Pushkin's subversive understanding of the nature of tyranny has been addressed by many subsequent Russian poets, including Joseph Brodsky. Instead of the Prince we have Stalin, the despot as paranoid, whose 'passion for survival' in a political landscape made oppressive by his doings leads him to destroy all those who might possibly pose a threat to his rule.

Pushkin's upas tree poem is a parable about despotism and domination, and how Russia's long history of hard-nosed dealings with its neighbours has poisoned regional politics, a situation that, as we are reminded from time to time, continues to this day. It is also in the Russian Federation that we find a contemporary upas tree with tap-roots descending deep into the history of the industrial exploitation of nature as well as into the nature of political power. At the foot of the Putoran Mountains, between the Yenisei River and Taymyr Peninsula is the ancient geological formation called the Siberian Traps, the flood basalt remnant of the paroxysmal eruptions (Permian-Triassic extinction event) that palaeontologists believe caused the extinction of nearly all species on Earth about 250 million years ago: here is the city of Norilsk, the only major city in eastern Siberia that lies inside the Arctic Circle. The polar night in Norilsk lasts for six weeks in winter, blinding curtains of snow are commonplace, and the temperature can scrape around -50°C for weeks in January and February. Norilsk was founded at the end of the 1920s as the one of the main encampments of the boreal Gulag system: its nickel deposits are the most extensive in the world, and it also sits on vast seams of copper, platinum, cobalt, palladium and coal. Thousands of prisoners died there under the harsh conditions of forced labour, starvation, and intense cold in the years between 1935 and 1956, and detainees were being sent to the mines up to 1979: with a high accident rate and limited life expectancy it is still a dangerous place to work (and it appears in the top-ten list of the Blacksmith Institute's report on the Worst Polluted Places, 2007). Now the city is run by a company called Norilsk Nickel, which raises capital and trades in all the respectable places: it is a major player in the global extraction business. Norilsk (population 175 000) is still a closed city, a useful Soviet-era policy which has never been lifted in some places although you can apparently link up to their inhabitants on the web.

After sixty years of mining and smelting, it has become economically cost-effective to work the polluted soil around the mines in order to recuperate the heavy metals dispersed in the initial tailings. That can only be described as a death-star vision of recycling. Norilsk's heavy metal smelter—where the ores are melted in what Blake would have called 'the Furnaces of Affliction'—is the largest in the world, with an annual atmospheric blow-off of many tons of cadmium, copper, lead, nickel, arsenic, selenium and zinc as well as several radio-isotopes. Within thirty miles of the nickel smelter, according to a CNN report in 2007, there is not a single living Siberian larch, the only tree that survives in the taiga. The name of the smelter is Nadezhda ('Hope').

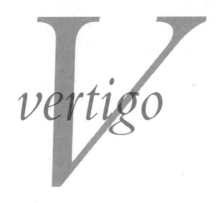

Stendhal's Syndrome

OR, HOW ART CAN MAKE YOU LOSE YOUR WITS

Well before the nineteenth century, there were travellers on the poorly maintained roads of Europe, most of them rich Englishmen doing the Grand Tour with their tutors. Then, around the time of the French Revolution (or a little before it), when the 'true voice of feeling' was loosed on the world by Jean-Jacques Rousseau, Laurence Sterne and a young German writer called Wilhelm von Goethe, figures we would recognise as modern travellers, might be spied moving on the roads. Hard on their heels came a certain Napoleon—arch romantic, poet and wit—who insisted on visiting the last-named author in Weimar during one of his whirlwind campaigns in the east, a copy of his novella about a love-sick suicide in his pocket.

And it was in Napoleon's entourage that a young man from Grenoble, Marie-Henri Beyle, known through his writings as Stendhal, earned his spurs. He made his first acquaintance with Italy in 1800, when he crossed as a dragoon in the army of liberation over the Grand Saint-Bernard pass to fight the Austrians, and it was to remain his country of predilection. And he 'fell', as he put it, when Napoleon's glorious career came to an end in 1814. After the Treaty of Fontainebleau he settled for a while in Milan, and later in life was to be French consul at Trieste and Cività Vecchia. Many of his greatest books are set in Italy, including his autobiography *The Life of Henry Brulard* (Brulard was one of his many aliases), which opens with the writer looking out from the Janiculum Hill with 'the whole of Rome [...] from the ancient Appian Way with the ruins of its tombs and aqueducts to the magnificent garden of the Pincio, built by the French, spread out before me'. He travelled widely, briefly visited Spain, spent two years as a quartermaster in northern Germany (whence the pen-name), and was in Russia with the Grande Armée, on that infamous journey to Moscow and back that turned into a horrendous saga of frostbite and starvation and lost lives. He went to London three times, and even contributed articles to English-language journals on the cultural life of Paris. Much of Stendhal's authority as a writer derives from his assumed persona as a guide who knows (and shows us) how to absorb what we experience in and of the rapidly changing world. That was the nineteenth century's principal novelty. Accordingly, he liked to pepper his French with anglicisms; and was one of the first writers to popularise the use of the word 'tourist' in French. (The one truly epic trip he never wrote about was the terrible, gruelling, inglorious retreat from Moscow.)

It was on one of his visits to Italy in 1811 that Stendhal brought the swoon into literature. Visiting the Basilica of Santa Croce in Florence, he found a monk to let him into the chapel where he could sit on a genuflection stool, tilt his head back and take in the prospect of Volterrano's fresco of the Sibyls without interruption.

The pleasure was keen. 'I was already in a kind of ecstasy', he writes, 'by the idea of being in Florence, and the proximity of the great men whose tombs I had just seen. Absorbed in contemplating sublime beauty, I saw it close-up—I touched it, so to speak. I had reached that point of emotion where the heavenly sensations of the fine arts meet passionate feeling. As I emerged from Santa Croce, I had palpitations (what they call an attack of the nerves in Berlin); the life went out of me, and I walked in fear of falling.' This vasovagal syncope prodrome (to give it its neurological name) was something he had observed many times of himself: 'when a thought takes too strong a hold of me in the middle of the street,' he writes in chapter 29 of his autobiography, 'I fall down.'

While contemplating artistic beauty he had created a new perspective for himself: a sense of depth so intense he lost his footing, and fell into it. Others would call it vertigo; and sure enough Stendhal is one of the cases written up in W. G. Sebald's four-part book *Schwindel. Gefühle* (translated into English as *Vertigo* although it divides what is one compound noun in German— *Schwindelgefühle* or 'feelings of dizziness'—into its punning component parts, one of which suggests that a swindle or trick is being played through a blatant display of feeling).

There were to be many cases resembling Stendhal's experience in the nineteenth century—the hypersensitive Marcel Proust had constant attacks of the vapours (and asthma) on his via dolorosa through *A la Recherche du Temps Perdu*, and Dostoevsky is known to have become terribly agitated when he saw the famous painting of the dead Christ by Hans Holbein the Younger in Basle (and made his pregnant wife fear he was going to have one of his epileptic fits). In his first Duino Elegy, the German poet Rainer Maria Rilke wrote: 'beauty is nothing but the beginning of terror, which we are still just able to endure, and are so awed because it serenely disdains to annihilate us'. Roland Barthes' term for it was 'la petite mort'. Great art is a threat. It can harbour a hidden violence so forceful that impressionable people forget who and where they are. Rilke's definition of beauty is perhaps more exactly a definition of its more masculine counterpart, 'the sublime'—the sensation that comes over us when we grasp the transcendent force of the sacred looming into the cultural. And as Rilke suggests, the sensation is followed by relief at being saved from annihilation by something greater than mere propositional language.

Philosophers were getting in on the act, too. Immanuel Kant in his *Critique of Judgement* hypothesised that the contemplation of aesthetically stimulating objects induces 'a rapidly alternating repulsion and attraction produced by one and the same object. The point of excess for the imagination [...] is like an abyss in which it fears to lose itself.' Nineteenth-century aesthetics abandoned the classical idea of imitation and took on the notion that contemplating an object was a self-activity experienced as an attribute of the object. This involuntary emotional projection was called *Einfühlung*: it is the German word that was brought into English as 'empathy'.

Stendhal's syndrome isn't one of the disorders listed in the latest edition of the *Diagnostic and Statistical Manual of Mental Disorders (DSM V)*, but in view of the nosological inventiveness shown by the editors of that manual in recent years it may well be just a matter of time. In 1989, Graziella Magherini, an enterprising psychiatrist at the Santa Maria Nuova hospital in Florence published a book of case studies *La Sindrome di Stendhal* on the 106 visitors who had been treated as emergencies and even hospitalised in her department in the previous decade. Their symptoms included dizzy spells, palpitations, hallucinations, disorientation, loss of identity and physical exhaustion. Precipitating factors were 'an impressionable personality, the stress of travel and the encounter with a city like Florence haunted by ghosts of the great, death and the perspective of history'.

The treatment was simple. It involved getting out of Italy as fast as possible and back to mundane reality. In honour of Stendhal's visit to the city she dubbed this phenomenon 'Stendhal's syndrome'.

But is Stendhal's syndrome anything new? In religious times, pilgrims often recorded a sense of exaltation on arriving in Rome, the *caput mundi*: the experience of feeling a little bit lighter (in all senses) once they get to their destination is an experience common to pilgrims across the world, from Mecca to Santiago de Compostela. After all, a prolonged journey is an archetypal experience: we enjoy reading travel literature because it allows us a vicarious share in the author's conviction of being on a quest. Goethe's famous Italian journey of 1786—away from his civil servant's desk—is one such example; he thought he would have been 'a lost man' if he hadn't been able to see Italy when he did. And there is nothing new either about the urge to sightsee: the Greeks were doing it in antiquity, and Herodotus and Callimachus had already tried to meet the demand for tourist attractions ('mirabilia') by listing the Seven Wonders around the shores of the Mediterranean. Even in those days travellers had a talent for coming back with useless souvenirs.

In view of its awestruck nature it could have been predicted that Stendhal's syndrome would find most florid and toponymic expression among religious travellers. In an article in the *British Journal of Psychiatry* in 2000, a team of psychiatrists at the Kfer Shaul Mental Health Centre in Jerusalem reported on an acute psychotic state dubbed 'Jerusalem syndrome'. Jerusalem, they write, is a city regarded in terms of 'the holy, the historical and the heavenly' by adherents of three of the world's religions, who are often blind and deaf to the politically divided, noisy and bustling modern city around them. They are after the transcendental, which has always been inimical to the pull of gravity. Jerusalem, after all, is the most potent metaphor in the history of the world. Tourists suffering from 'psychotic decompensation'—all of them—are referred to their facility at Kfer Shaul: that makes for an average of about 100 patients a year, forty of whom require admission. The psychiatrists distinguish three types of patients: those with pre-existing problems, usually pathological identification with a character or idea, those with borderline personality disorders, and previously normal persons experiencing a short-lived acute psychotic episode, similar in many ways to Stendhal's syndrome but manifested by a desire to sing psalms out loud, wrap themselves in pristine hotel bed-linen or deliver loud sermons to passers-by in the city's holy places. Such patients, the authors discovered, have 'an idealistic subconscious image of Jerusalem'. Recovery was generally spontaneous on leaving the city.

In his autobiography *Memories, Dreams, Reflections* Carl Gustav Jung describes how in 1949, by then an old man, he decided to go to Rome, something he had wished to do all his life but had put off, fearing the emotional impact of encountering the heart of Europe's ancient imperial structure. Pompeii, which he had visited many years earlier, had exerted an effect which 'had very nearly exceeded [his] powers of receptivity'. The day he went to buy his ticket from the travel agent in Zurich he fainted. 'After that, the plans for a trip to Rome were once and for all laid aside.' Jung was never to see the Eternal City because of his idealistic subconscious image of it. Sigmund Freud, who had perhaps played a role in priming his former acolyte's imaginative receptivity to the idea of Rome, had a similar lifelong thing about Athens. Which shows that one way to avoid an experience is not to have it at all. On the other hand, not paying attention to your subconscious can get you into a lot of bother: embassies in India and the insurance company Europ Assistance (a subsidiary of the Triestine insurance company Assicurazioni Generali that Franz Kafka once worked for) are perfectly familiar with young Europeans who, in mystical transport, are found intoning unknown liturgies while climbing the stairs to their New Delhi hotels on their knees, and have to be repatriated as emergency cases. Japanese tourists to Paris apparently suffer from a condition known (in Japan) as Paris syndrome—the terrible sense of failure at not being able to visit all of the French capital's listed museums in the allotted time.

It occurred to me, thinking about these toponymic conditions (and realising I'd treated some of these Japanese tourists myself when I worked at the American Hospital of Paris in 1985), that the aforementioned Israeli doctors had clearly never read the Talmud of Babylon, which states that Jerusalem is one of the 'things which were created before the world'. A city that existed before history—now that is a concept worth wrestling with. It ought to give anyone a flutter of Jerusalem syndrome.

Actually, it's quite unsettling when people you assume to be sensible turn out to be histrionic at heart. The journalist Louis Inturissi, in a hilarious piece for *The New York Times* in 1988, suggested that many Americans who come down with Stendhal's Syndrome have simply OD'd on art. Like the Japanese tourists in Paris, they have to 'do' Florence, Rome and Naples in two days, and it almost kills them. Moreover, works of the imagination can sometimes pall dreadfully. Dr Johnson, who was a most reluctant traveller (James Boswell dragged him all the way up to the Western Isles of Scotland, in those days a monumental trek and not a journey undertaken for pleasure), suggested that 'the use of travelling is to regulate imagination by reality'. But the reality encountered on travelling can overwhelm even the best-regulated imagination. I've personally experienced Jakarta Syndrome, which is a kind of sinking feeling in the centre of a major Asian city of at least ten million souls when you realise there is almost nothing on offer for adoration except the atrium of a modern five-star hotel.

At the other end of the spectrum from the art attack described by Stendhal is another kind of condition. Inturissi calls it Mark Twain Malaise, a cynical mood that overcomes travellers and leaves them totally unimpressed with anything Unesco has on its universal heritage list. In his account *The Innocents Abroad*, one of the best-selling travel books ever published, Twain, who takes some delight in lampooning the grandiose travel accounts of his contemporaries, was impudent enough to suggest that when he saw Leonardo's *Last Supper* in the dilapidated monastery of Santa Maria delle Grazie in Milan his first thought had been that the copies he had seen back home were so much better than the orig- inal. (He was right of course; the painting was in a terrible state until very recently, largely because Leonardo *knowingly* chose to used flawed materials in his stucco.) 'I am willing to believe', he wrote, 'that the eye of the practised artist can rest upon the Last Supper and renew a lustre where only a hint of it is left, supply a tint that has faded away, restore an expression that is gone [...] But I cannot work this miracle. Can those other uninspired visitors do it, or do they only happily imagine they do?' Years before Twain, John Ruskin, mistrustful of the new-fangled enterprise of tourism, had declared that he didn't find romance in Venice, which is 'simply a heap of ruins trodden underfoot', but nevertheless might have wondered if the publication of his book *The Stones of Venice* had had something to do with the steep rise in romance-seekers to the watery city thereafter.

More recently, in what might be called his anticipatory memoir *Nothing to be Frightened Of*, Julian Barnes remembered Stendhal's account of his intense experience of the Florentine fresco. Intrigued, he did some research on the original diary entries concerning the writer's trip to Italy and found no mention of the arty faint. That day—26 September 1811—Stendhal records that he had been dead tired, and his feet were swollen and pinching because of his new boots—'a little sensation that would prevent God from being admired in the midst of His glory'; but as he gamely continued, 'I overlooked it in front of the picture of *Limbo*.' It was his servant who had told him to take a look at the Sibyls anyway. He records being all aflutter at the experience, but there is nothing about swooning on the way out of Santa Croce.

So there we have it: there is no Stendhal syndrome. Stendhal appears never to have had the experience he wrote up in his trav- elogue. Or at least if he did have it he had it as Beyle, and wrote it up as Stendhal. It was a self-performance that turned an apparently random date in the life of Henri Beyle into a spectacle in which the phenomenon *Stendhal* could be shared with others: in a word, a work of art.

We all react imaginatively to great art in the belief that, in a true fellowship of feeling, subject and object merge. That idea is as old as Plato, who still had some qualms about the ritualistic nature of aesthetic objects and the obliterating violence of inspiration (which we acknowledge when we talk about being 'struck' by a work of art). Art can be so powerful we forget its unpredictability or even the reality it is supposed to represent, and faint like Mary at the Cross. All those scenes were familiar too to that wizard Stendhal, who fostered a cult of spontaneity but whose novels insist on reminding us that in the world of desire a little water is always needed to prime a pump.

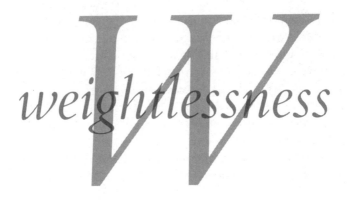

weightlessness

The War of Eye and Ear

ON THE SENSES CONSIDERED AS PERCEPTUAL SYSTEMS

'…he who strains to listen doesn't see.'
Walter Benjamin, letter to Gerhard Scholem

1

Since the dawn of what Norbert Elias called 'the process of civilisation', sight has held an undisputed place as the most estimable of the senses. Asked what he had been born for, one of the earliest philosophers, Anaxagoras, replied: 'For seeing.' According to Heraclitus, the enigmatic philosopher who taught that humanity was an organic extension of the Logos, 'eyes are better informers than ears'. Plato was every bit as philoscopic. That cornerstone of Western philosophy, Aristotle's writings, opens with the assertion: 'most of all, we esteem the sense of sight'. Hippocrates, the father of medicine, a bookish authority for later generations of physicians, also pleaded for the evidence of things seen. Although the ancient understanding of seeing—as a kind of effluence of the person, or what is called *extramission*—has little in common with the mathematics of modern optics, by the fifth century BC visual acuity and the attributes of knowledge were already one: the Greek verb *theorein* means 'to contemplate'.

So when Greek ideas were rediscovered at the beginning of what we call the Renaissance it wasn't just those troublesome anti-thetical terms from the pre-Socratic era, especially that conceptual pair light-dark, the former being 'noble' (like male, dry and right), the latter 'ignoble' (like female, wet and left), that were given a new lease of life. The mind's eye beheld the world afresh: knowledge was once more analogous to vision. But less and less did things have a quality that corresponded to the eye. Leon Battista Alberti's wooden frame for establishing a perspectival construct of objects in space, of which Albrecht Dürer in a famous woodcut demonstrates the use, has tellingly been called an 'optical scalpel'. The greatest figure of the Renaissance, Leonardo da Vinci, restricted his studies to the domain of what he called *sperienza*, by which he meant chiefly visual experience. He already understood the new epistemology. The eye was a potentate, ordering the universe and rectifying jumble and clutter in accordance with the rules of perspective. Knowledge was predicated on things being made visible, for darkness was where ignorance brooded. Want, famine and destitution throve in the dark, and only the light of reason could bring salvation from such primordial terrors. As Jean Star-obinski tells us, 'Metaphors of light triumphing over darkness [...] were to be found everywhere in the period leading up to 1789.' The French Revolution hardly even had to announce itself as the advent of light, a new dawn for humankind. It was modernity's solar myth, its own beatification.

By the early nineteenth century, imagination had thrown its lot behind seeing—we can visualise even with our eyes closed (OED: 'visualise: to construct a visual image in the mind'), but nobody has ever been known to *audibilise, gustatise, olfactorise* or *tactualise*. No sense except the visual has a geometry, which extends into space, while the other senses work intensively in time.

We enjoy the other senses for their adjectival qualities. For instance, there must have been a brief period at the beginning of the modern era, to judge from Rabelais' wonderful lists of body parts restyled as foods in *Gargantua and Pantagruel*, when the gustatory was king, and the mouth, as in the Bible, still the route to true understanding. 'Open your mouth, and eat what I give you', the prophet Ezekiel is instructed. In French, knowledge (savoir) and taste (saveur) are still recognisably the same word. One famous chapter in Rabelais' second book even takes place inside Pantagruel's oversized maw: Larynx and Pharynx are two large cities 'like Rouen and Nantes', and the cause of the plague turns out to be the foul vapours resulting from the giant eating too much garlic sauce. The culture of early modern Europe revelled in its fleshiness: starved of material goods, it generated Goliardic fantasies of sated bodies. But the solidly incarnate person didn't survive the sixteenth century, and Gluttony, alone among the seven major vices, has become an even more venial sin in our secular age.

Shakespeare suggests what happened, in his retelling of Menenius Agrippa's ancient fable of the dispute between the members and the stomach, in the opening lines of *Coriolanus*:

There was a time, when all the body's members
Rebell'd against the belly; thus accus'd it:
That only like a gulf it did remain
I'th'midst o'th' body, idle and unactive,
Still cupboarding the viand, never bearing
Like labour with the rest, where th'other instruments
Did see, and hear, devise, instruct, walk, feel,
And, mutually participate, did minister
Unto the appetite and affection common
Of the whole body [...]

2

Now eye motifs so imperiously govern our metaphors for understanding we scarcely notice our minds have gone the way our vision took them. Enlightenment has become a bedazzlement, if not a blinding, and entire eras that went before ours are left to moulder in that dungeon called the Dark Ages. The closer you look at it the more the life of Francis Bacon, that PR man for modern lighting fixtures, was a pretty dark thing, and the early medieval period in Europe actually one of great intellectual vitality, especially around the Mediterranean when the power and brilliance of Islam were at their height: the medical school at Salerno, which provided the model of medical education for all the great medieval universities of Europe, was founded just after the turn of the first millennium.

It doesn't take a sociologist, or even a historian of science, to tell us that human relations are dominated, as never before, by sight. The empirical philosophers contended that we cannot know why things are as they are, and have to content ourselves describing what we cannot help believing any more than we can help seeing: they put perception in a cave where everything resembles events in the external world but there is no means of verifying the degree of resemblance. In the empiricist hall of mirrors you *see* what is meant, bring things into *focus*, throw *light* on the matter. Even Shakespeare joins the chorus, with his famous line in Hamlet: 'In the mind's eye, Horatio.' The brooding inner eye, cyclopean rather than binocular, can be found in St Paul and Plato too: the metaphor invites us to contemplate being spied out of our wits. In what infinitely regressive mental organ is the mind's mind's eye? Soon we suspect that there's something rather chimerical about our perceptions, especially about the kind of seeing that confers bliss, as in Teilhard de Chardin's notion of the cosmos aiming at 'the elaboration of ever more perfect eyes'. (So what happened to that other property of eyes which brims so often from Dante's in the *Purgatario*?)

In spite of its genial anticlericalism, Rabelais' humanism was disregarded during the eighteenth century, the age of the lights: Voltaire thought his writings a mere impertinence. Victor Hugo, a century later in the age of *l'homme moyen sensuel*, couldn't make head nor tail of them. All their images of bodily life, those fantastic catalogues of eating, drinking, copulation and defecation, had lost what Mikhail Bakhtin, in his famous study of Rabelais and his world, assures us was their regenerating power. For the *philosophes* they were aspects of the crass superstition of the agrarian age, mere grotesquery. Knowledge had already begun to explode in the age of Rabelais, when Europe moved out to colonize the utopias its pious thinkers had prepared for it; the Enlightenment applied techniques of hygiene to the mind in order to disburden it of the medieval era's fantastic profusion of theories and interpretations.

Memory was devalued in favour of lexicography. Knowledge had become a topology.

Yet the stories that Rabelais took from folk culture, when penury and hunger belonged to the category of natural things, were fearless: terror was something comic, to be repulsed by laughter. Rabelais' exuberant books remove themselves from the fixed view of medieval thinking: he dares the reader to be taken by surprise, to play with words, to venture into the wide world though it be, as Erich Auerbach added, 'at his own peril'. Laughter is the mark of our humanity, wrote Rabelais. Nothing else we do is so richly ambivalent about standing out from the crowd: a liberal laughing *with*, an illiberal laughing *at*—or as Nietzsche described it: 'being *schadenfroh* but with a good conscience'. Laughter is involuntary and reciprocal: that's why it's infectious. And we end up laughing so much we seem to be sobbing: 'If you read as I wrote it, for mere amusement, we are both more deserving of forgiveness than that great rabble of quality statesmen, facilitators, agony aunts, soul dissectors, dog heads, hypocrites, careerists, members of the Church of Merited and Blessed Health, moralists in white coats, and other such sects of people, who have disguised themselves like maskers, to deceive the world.'

3

That world of cheekiness is pretty much alien to us: one distinguished contemporary historian, Norman Davies, even asked in his great history of Europe whether Rabelais wasn't the last European to be truly human. Lucien Febvre suggests that the entire epoch is lost to us: 'the sixteenth century did not see first, it heard and smelled, it sniffed the air and caught sounds'. And it's not just the loss of the lower senses that horrify people; it's the insight that in the future we might lose what George Steiner called 'real presence'—being embodied, the dependability of material realities, face-to-face dealings with others, genuine community.

Sight is now our metonym for the raw feel of perception in general, for no other sense offers such mastery. It is the only one that never loses out from being at a distance: indeed knowledge at a sighted remove is often *foreknowledge*. It is the expanded sense of Marshall McLuhan's famous Gutenberg galaxy where the margins, chapters, linearity and punctuation of the book supply the structural model for a city divided into parks, districts, roads and bureaucracies. Yet sight's nobility and universality, as Descartes called them—and his *cogito* that couldn't reasonably doubt itself is essentially specular, a mirroring back to the self of the assertion that a self should be—are deficient: looking and seeing (for the former has to be learned before you can accomplish the latter) provide possibilities for action, but require the support of more vulgar mediators, especially the hand, that Jeeves of an organ, to maintain a commerce with the world. It is the other senses that do sight's living.

Our world, just in case you hadn't noticed, is organised around images. As Georg Simmel wrote in *The Metropolis*, 'interpersonal relationships in big cities are distinguished by a marked preponderance of the eye over the activity of the ear'. This is particularly evident in medicine, which is a parade of bodies, though the exhibits we get to examine, as more or less trained interpreters, seem to be part of an ever less embodied reality. Sight is pervasive, overpowering, indiscriminate. 'One can terrify with one's eye, not with one's ear or nose', noticed Ludwig Wittgenstein. I can't be alone in finding eerie parallels between the closed circuit panopticons of our cities and the ability of scopic technologies to render us transparent. In order to become an image a body must surrender its matter. Images are *simulacra*. They are a kind of consolation for never getting to grips with things at all, an invitation to the coldest kind of theatricality as well as a desperate expression of the need for human warmth.

Perhaps that's one reason why patients flock to the hot springs and temples of alternative practitioners: they simply can't cope with the shame of seeing themselves vivisected on celluloid or pixilated. They want to feel themselves living, to participate in a notion of health as old as Pythagoras' harmonies, though they know weightlessness is the fate of a world where knowledge has been drilled to see through every solid body, including their own. In the age of virtual reality, Narcissus is the essential classical model for psychic survival, though Narcissus knows, when the round of self-adoration fails to function, that his ethereally infinite ego is but a purely formal unity of representations. Self-love is anything but sufficient unto itself: as Shakespeare's plays show us, time and again, self-love is prisoner to its enslavement by significant others. Venturing out of his private oasis to tread the jungle of the streets, Narcissus may even recall that street-corner cameras find their philosophical origin in Jeremy Bentham's ideas for the modern penitentiary.

It may be a problem for the medical profession, too. Bulging with the amputated minds that make medical method so powerful, but limit it too, doctors can hardly escape another, perhaps more disturbing tension. Is the profession pledged to the eye, or to the ear? After all, everything starts with listening. It is, one might say, an attitude prior even to care and concern. The descant of the ear is a reminder of medicine's archaic past. Unlike the imperialising eye, the ear is humble. It has to be; it is a servant. In Latin, 'obedience' (*obedientia*) is derived from the verb for 'lending ear to' (*obaudire*). The old-fashioned verbal command 'hearken' carries the same charge in English. 'The ear is much slower in comprehension than the eye, far less avid of novelty, and far more appreciative of rhythmical repetition', wrote W. H. Auden. The Austrian poet Rainer Maria Rilke, who influenced Auden much in mid-life, defined his own life as a poet, in which inspiration came to him like occasional rain to a desert plant, as 'days of enormous obedience'. Of course, demagogues and dictators adore people who are all ears: they run their regimes on the principle that there should be no gap between command and action. In the doctor's office, however, it is precisely the person invested with the power—the power to heal—who is obliged to listen.

Sound is bound: to duration, and other kinds of trespass—it has to wait, it has to make room, it has to be patient.

Appropriately enough, the ear is often considered *the* religious organ, at least in iconographic representations of the Annunciation: the Virgin Mary conceives through hers. The infant Gargantua, in Rabelais' book, gets dislodged from his mother's womb after she takes a purgative for eating too much tripe, slips into a vein, and gets born through hers—and you might almost say that the modern novel has been the afterbirth. In Psalm 40, David thanks God for having so deeply 'hollowed out his ear'. Why should he say that? Because you can't hear anything with your throat; or as the poet W. S. Graham wrote in a fine couplet: 'the ear says more / than any tongue'. The ear is hope's conduit. People who listen hard often close their eyes. In his commentary on the *Sefer Bahir*, Gershom Scholem tells us that the ear is the image of Aleph, 'and Aleph is the first of all letters; more than that, Aleph is the precondition for the existence of all the letters'.

4

In fact, the ear is as close as medicine gets, or might want to get, to religion. The story in *Acts of the Apostles* about what happened at the Pentecost is usually interpreted as authority for the gibberish of the Unknown Tongue. The more garbled the words the greater the proof of divine inspiration. That's the practice (there's no theory), though I must confess the original recording of James Joyce reading *Anna Livia Plurabelle* is probably the only bit of pentecostalism I've ever listened to with enjoyment, and it surely doesn't qualify, since it was long premeditated, delivered chapter by chapter to a small magazine, and written up in a gloriously theatrical universal language by an Irish philologist with a perfect English ear (and a deep love of Rabelais). But let me turn the rhetorical tables. Since hearing is an existential possibility in the act of talking itself, why shouldn't the incident at Pentecost actually be a story about reception?—a miracle of listening with ears, not speaking in tongues. For ten minutes, or even a bit longer, the curse of Babel is lifted by a readiness to listen.

I suspect most doctors have had a few Pentecostal experiences in their careers. Nothing spectacular, no flash of light on the Damascus Road—just a slight change of tone and register. Enough to prove that simultaneous translation really can happen, even when patient and doctor do speak the same language. For if Hume's scepticism teaches us that we cannot even know the world exists, then knowledge is the wrong way to approach it. 'The world is to be accepted; as the presentness of other minds is not to be known, but acknowledged', writes Stanley Cavell in his essay *The Avoidance of Love: A Reading of King Lear*.

It seems to me, however, that ear and eye are fated not to be at peace. Not even now that the body has been rehabilitated. Especially not now. Ours is supposedly an age of body language, body image, body art, body consciousness even. The 1960s made a revolution out of liberating the body, as if its reality, despite those lines in Genesis about its being the very first object of knowledge to enter consciousness, had just become apparent. Another odd thing about the rehabilitated body: it only lets itself go under controlled conditions. The truth is that our carnival is nothing like Rabelais'. Ours is the cult of the machine for living, not the carnival of the whole body. The price of the ticket for our ability to manipulate material things—and our lives are inconceivably more comfortable than those of Shakespeare's kings—has been surrender of our social mutuality; everything that lives on trust. (Not that trust disappears, for no human system can operate without it: it just becomes weaker and more etiolated.) But what can social beings do for conviviality when the eye, that most enlightened of tyrants, politely but firmly refuses to know anything at all about a place called Babel, where CCTV cameras have been fitted to the top of the tower? These days, according to the eye, we have escaped the age of fear and faith. We are autonomous, and that's no laughing matter.

The deep problem with the eye is this: it got to boast about being noble only by blinding itself to the totality of experience. Shakespeare's *King Lear* turns on that very paradox. What we see is not the whole of what there is to see; what is seen is only a segment of what may potentially be known; and so the truth of our experience contrives to hide from us. As Marshall McLuhan writes, 'Probably any medieval person would be puzzled at our idea of looking through something. He would assume that the reality looked through at us, and that by contemplation we bathed in the divine light, rather than looked at it.' That's what that life-long troublemaker William Blake was getting at in *Milton* when, in accordance with his conviction that imagination is the *ratio*—'the most precious square of sense'—holding the perceptive faculties in harmony, he described man prosthetically extended or 'outed' to his sense organs. In his version of the whole man every faculty is equally impoverished in its extension:

> The Eye of Man, a little narrow orb, clos'd up & dark,
> Scarcely beholding the Great Light, conversing with the ground:
> The Ear, a little shell, in small volutions shutting out
> True Harmonies, & comprehending great as very small [...]

Our civilisation is actually founded on an explicit *restriction* of cognition, on aspect-blindness. As the veil of ignorance lifts, totality recedes ever further out of sight; indeed other aspects of experience may become inaccessible.

Some of us, however, are still smelling our way to Dover. Far from having escaped the age of fear, the eye has stumbled on Shakespeare's cupboard of viand. The more the eye insists on watchfulness, installs ophthalmic surrogates and prostheses wherever it can, and generally believes like an American in the gospel of prevention, the more its vision of the world seems partial, if not paranoid. For its gothic discovery is this: the body, that blackguard in the kitchens of a solid bourgeois mansion, that ruffian on the stairs, is some kind of Mr Hyde plotting to rob it of its integrity. And suddenly what seemed our biggest investment, our bit of plastic, our self-project, our adored machine for living, turns out to have a mind of its own. Smooth skin on the outside, Old Adam in.

What name should we give to it, then—enemy?

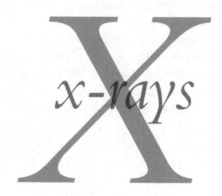

x-rays

Under the Magic Mountain

FROM THE TB SANATORIUM TO MEDICAL TOURISM

An Alpine regime

In his influential commentary on Thomas Mann's novel *The Magic Mountain* (1924), which appeared just a few years after the novel itself, the scholar Hermann Weigand called it 'the epic of disease'.

We need to define terms. Mann's novel is more accurately characterised as the epic of *a* disease, tuberculosis, a major disease that has accompanied humans throughout their history, at least since they started building and settling in cities. It is also, in the broader sense, an epic of *illness*—an ambitious attempt to show how the condition of being ill (a more subjective category than disease) was experienced in a particular culture at a particular time in its history.

In the nineteenth century, and not just in Germany, being tubercular was associated with being 'interesting'—and making yourself interesting is the primordial Romantic impulse. The main character in the novel adopts the sick role with a sense of exaltation—and at times even election—that goes back to transcendental idealism and the supposition, first expressed by the poet Novalis, that illness might be 'the means to a higher synthesis'. It is unsettling, then, that when seen from the 'flatland' (a code-word in the novel for ordinary existence) the same character comes across as a malinger who has jacked in his career in order to enjoy an institutionally coddled life on the mountain top where he will become a virtuoso in selfhood. In *mere* selfhood, one is tempted to add.

As Thomas Mann himself suggested, his hero Hans Castorp—a kind of dreamy Candide whose face, as with Voltaire's famous fictional character, is 'the index of his mind'—is on a somewhat paradoxical quest: he has to pass through illness to rediscover the ethics of normal life itself. That is a search we are all familiar with, one way or another: the magic mountain is no longer a retreat or social height; it is the familiar landscape, at least in the developed world, of a technological Eden with no more onerous a task than organising our entire lives. On the bottom rung of all this reorganising is a medical sociologist's platitude: the healthier we become the more medicine we demand. In the words of Nikolas Rose: 'like Hans Castorp upon his Magic Mountain, our stay in the sanatorium is not limited to a brief and terminable episode of illness. It is a sentence without limits and without walls, in which, apparently of our own free will and with the best of intentions on all sides, our existence has become bound to the ministrations and adjudications of medical expertise.'

When Mann began his novel, tuberculosis was at a significant juncture in its history: the discovery of the visible effects associated with an unknown type of electromagnetic radiation, X-rays, on the cusp of the twentieth century, had made it possible to detect with some accuracy early active pulmonary forms of the disease. Medicine's therapeutic capacities, however, lagged decades behind its diagnostic accuracy: it was only after the Second World War that effective antibacterial treatments emerged for TB. But treatment is lengthy and not always well tolerated, and patients tend to stop taking their treatment on the first signs of remission. This abets the development of resistant forms. Even today, despite the newer drugs available to treat it, containment campaigns in many developing countries have only been partially successful and TB remains a major public health problem, not least in its multidrug-resistant forms: it is thought there are now more cases of TB worldwide than at any time in history. It has been calculated that fully about one-third of the global population has been exposed to the bacillus (although only a percentage of those exposed go on to develop the disease).

The Magic Mountain takes us to one of the few therapeutic options open to the better-heeled European patient of that time: a 'change of air' in the spa or sanatorium—what the Italians call *villegiatura*.

Going up into a mountain retreat was one of the growth sectors of Switzerland's economy in the nineteenth century. From about 1860 to 1940, an Alpine regime of rest and rich food was thought to provide the best chance for recovery from TB, and for the body to work its healing 'wisdom'. It was a policy that certainly isolated patients with active disease (who were spreading the infection through coughing or sneezing) from the general population, but it made for local environments that had high circulating levels of airborne bacilli. Indeed, the atmosphere of the Haus Berghof, on the Davos plateau, to which Mann in the opening pages of his novel propels Hans Castorp, is not quite as wholesome as it might seem. The thin mountain air, much as in the *Bergfilme* (mountain films) that were popular in the years of Weimar Republic and later promoted by the Nazis as the German answer to the Western movie, proves to be anything but pure and clean; it turns out to be a narcotic, heady and disorientating.

Hans, who has just passed his engineering exams in Hamburg, is travelling up from the 'flatland' into the mountains to visit his cousin Joachim Ziemssen, an aspiring soldier with established TB. He plans to go for a three-week holiday and ends up staying seven years: the Berghof wins him over in the way people sent out to the European colonies used to be accused of 'going native'. In this rarefied atmosphere snow falls all year round and all days become 'a continuous present, an identity, and everlastingness'. It is where the consumptives are confined, lying out in blankets on rattan deck-chairs to breathe the glacial air by day—the famous *Liegekur*—and retiring to their rooms to cough out their lungs at night. They live 'horizontally', as Joachim remarks to Hans.

This society in exile is a circle of the living dead or *moribundi*, yet to Hans its members seem frivolous and even disobligingly superficial: the foppish Herr Albin likes to upset his fellow diners by pressing a revolver to his temple and Hermine Kleefeld, a leading light of the Half-Lung Club—a select bunch of patients who have undergone a surgical pneumothorax procedure to collapse temporarily the affected lung—whistles at Hans 'from somewhere inside'. When not being slothful and eating copious amounts of food—a typical gourmet meal would comprise a chaud-froid of chicken garnished with crayfish and stoned cherries followed by ice-cream and pastries in spun-sugar baskets—they indulge in an easy-going eroticism: the high-minded Hans at the outset of his stay is offended by the amorous sounds of the Russian couple in the next room '[whose] game had passed quite frankly over into the bestial'. In general, opting for the sick-role on the magic mountain seems to open the door on a life of constant good spirits and endless fun, not lucidity and depth about the human condition.

Perhaps being afflicted with TB, as all those nineteenth-century operas proclaim, was indeed an aphrodisiac.

How Hans becomes what he is

Improbable as it might seem to us, its present readers, *The Magic Mountain* started out as a short story, in fact as a pendant to Mann's famous tale of disease and eroticism, *Death in Venice*. Mann had just finished work on that novella when he visited his wife Katia at Dr Jessen's Waldsanatorium in Davos in May and June 1912, and told one of his correspondents that he was working on a new project, a 'kind of countertext' to the Aschenbach story. Both offer a journey out of humdrum life into a luxury setting, and explore an existentially threatening situation subsequent to falling in love. But while Aschenbach is degraded by deciding that illness should be a reason for his not escaping the stricken city, Castorp, as Susan Sontag notes in *Illness as Metaphor*, is 'promoted'. 'The atmosphere was to be that strange mixture of death and lightheadedness I had found at Davos', wrote Mann, in his afterword to the novel. 'There was to be an ordinary hero, in conflict between bourgeois decorum and macabre adventure [...] Then the First

World War broke out. It did two things: put an immediate stop to my work on the book, and incalculably enriched its content at the same time.'

Like the steam train that transports Hans Castorp from Hamburg to the mountain, Mann himself was travelling from the comfortable patrician world of his upbringing to a more uncertain future: 'It takes place [...] in the old days, the days of the world before the Great War, in the beginning of which so much began that has scarcely yet left off beginning.' New possibilities are in the air (including having an upstart technician-engineer as the hero of a *Bildungsroman*, since it was still the case in imperial Germany that the professions open to the classically educated carried more prestige than engineering), but there is a certain reluctance about abandoning the old world altogether: bits of the old scenery loom out of the mist, deep chasms and bare peaks damp with mythic associations. And behind the old scenery we sense the self-consciously 'representative' writer who, on the outbreak of war, had been seduced by dreams of glorious service to the Fatherland, including what he called 'armed service with the pen'. After it, ruefully aware of his romantic penchant for pessimism and apocalypse, Mann had tried to find a place in a world run by technically competent yet unexceptional men like his Engineer. As late as 1918 he had published his bulky collection of polemical essays *Reflections of a Non-Political Man*, a passionate defence of Germany's participation in the war that goes so far as to identify his nation's cause with Kant's philosophy: as an arch-nationalist, he had argued against the liberal position of his own brother Heinrich, an enthusiastic Francophile. By 1922, Mann had completely changed his position, and gone public about his thinking on the matter—to the consternation of supporters and opponents alike. He had seen where it had led, all the talk of war as a rebirth of the spirit and an opportunity for Europe's moral regeneration. He was now a supporter of democratic republicanism, even of accommodation with what Bertolt Brecht called the 'bad new' things. *The Magic Mountain* is, over much of its length, an oblique account of his conversion.

An aspect of the 'good old' things that Mann insists on taking with him is the classic humanism of German culture, of which Johann Wolfgang von Goethe is the emblem and figurehead. It is in Goethe's early novella, *The Sorrows of Young Werther*, his story of an ardent soul and teenage suicide, that we find the origins of the descriptions of nature that break into Hans' stolid consciousness: 'Stupendous mountains encompassed me, abysses yawned at my feet, and cataracts fell headlong down before me; impetuous rivers rolled through the plain, and rocks and mountains resounded from afar.' Goethe's protagonists—notably the titular lead of his second novel, *Wilhelm Meister's Apprenticeship*—leave imprints all over Mann's novel: Hans is still ingenuous, in the sense that his native wit and intuition have not been educated out of him: early in the novel the narrator calls him 'this still unwritten page'. From being a rather feckless young man whose bedside reading material when he arrives at the Berghof is a technical book called *Ocean Steamships*, by the end of his stay he has acquired the kind of hermetic knowledge of 'the innermost force that holds the world together' that Goethe alludes to in the second book of Faust. In the spellbinding sphere of dreams and magic (*'Traum- und Zaubersphäre'*), another phrase from the same play, anything can happen: image can become reality and reality mere image, and a young man of promise can lose his soul.

Up on the mountain new cases arrive and old ones leave, some of them from the mortuary: the other sanatorium in the region, the Schatzalp, somewhat indelicately carts the bodies of its dead patients down in sledges during the winter. A death is never announced to other guests on the mountains: that would be considered an indecency. There are incoming messages from the flatland; there are even occasional visitors, including, in an amusing interlude, Hans' great-uncle (and guardian) James Tienappel, who pays a visit to the young man, after a year has lapsed, in order to persuade the lost sheep to return to Hamburg. Uncle James leaves in a hurry the next morning, apparently fearful of falling victim himself to the morbid charms of the Berghof. Uncle James 'had become inwardly aware', muses Hans later. 'After only a week up here, he would find everything down below wrong and out of place [...] It would seem to him unnatural to go to his office, instead of taking a prescribed walk after breakfast, and thereafter lying ritually wrapped, horizontal on a balcony.' The magic mountain is no prison, but its atmosphere has a terribly warping effect on common sense.

In this grandiose natural setting, Mann compels Castorp to tackle the opposing forces that so preoccupied him in his own career as a novelist: reason and irrationality, health and sickness, dynamism and pessimism, conscious will and unconscious impulse, West and East. Few novels of this length have a simpler narrative schema. And, of course, everything happens in sevens: the magical number is one of Mann's little jokes, and a major structural principle. It is evidence of Mann's skill as a novelist that his huge symbolic superstructure is able to nurture a society of characters and offer a genuine portrait of the age. It is one in which a middling young man is compelled to become a genius, at least about himself; and he is obliged to discover it through being ill. He lives his life as an individual even while expressing the life of his epoch.

Hans Castorp is a psychological man, sick to the degree that he is unable to find any authority in his upbringing that might give a sense of direction to his life. Indeed, *The Magic Mountain* explores ways in which self-knowledge might be made social, a reversal of the old understanding that knowing one's place comes about through obedience to family and community, to inherited tradition and the basic tenets of civility. Hans is, let us not forget, an orphan.

A negative epiphany

One morning Hofrat Behrens, the jovially cynical superintendent of the Berghof, tells Hans that he looks unwell—'*sine pecunia*', he adds twice, although he clearly has a vested interest in recruiting and retaining patients. Patients are free to leave the sanatorium, even against doctor's orders; Behrens merely shrugs his shoulders at the news of disloyal departure, and lets his arms clap against his sides: he enjoys predicting the date of their likely return 'to spend yet more earthly time at this pleasure resort'. Hans, as fascinated as he is alarmed, buys a state-of-the-art thermometer (which is 'like a jewel') and begins to record his temperature four times daily. In a rather innocent manner, Hans' adoption of routine fever-measuring foreshadows our more technically elaborate obsession with self-monitoring: the classic injunction 'know thyself' is something we do with numbers these days, not words.

Meanwhile, his cousin Joachim, the actual patient, chafes under his enforced leisure, and hankers to return to his flatland life in the army; Behrens—tongue not entirely in cheek—tells Hans that he'll make 'a better patient'.

On the point of embracing the possibility that he too might be ill, Hans meets the beguiling Russian, Clawdia Chauchat. With her blithe habit of slamming the dining room door, this 'Kirghiz-eyed' woman irritates him, and then starts to intrigue him. She is a free spirit who cares nothing for the kind of ordered reason that governs social conventions such as marriage, or even the proper running of the sanatorium. Her mysterious husband, who never turns up to reclaim her from the sanatorium, is an oil-engineer working at the centre of the then world oil industry in Daghestan, one of those 'heavenly rose-gardens' where Persia abuts on Russia in the eastern Caucasus. He is too busy siphoning the geological subconscious to appear in the novel: oil doesn't just fuel the modern economy and provide strategic objectives in time of war, it is the 'crude' stuff that energises the magic mountain and the life of its characters.

It will take Hans months—seven in fact—before he can work up the courage to address Clawdia. And such a troubling influence cannot go unchallenged. Hans meets the man who will play down her attractions: Ludovici Settembrini. Though Hans thinks he looks clownish on their first meeting, Settembrini proves to have a sobering influence on him. He requests to be his tutor, the humanistic pedagogue who will admonish Hans regularly for his waywardness and urge him to return to his professional life. Settembrini, the great defender of Western liberalism, has no truck with the supposition that illness might make a person more interesting. 'Disease and despair are often only forms of depravity.' Perfectly well people, he warns Hans, have even been known to insist on staying on the mountain.

But Clawdia and the East prevail, and they overcome Hans at the moment that we see through him with the help of Behren's X-ray machine—which Mann writes as a parody of the famous moment in 1896 when Wilhelm Röntgen first took an image of his wife's hand with his newly discovered invisible electromagnetic rays. The doctor concludes that Hans has a 'moist spot' on his lung and scars from a childhood infection, the same pronouncement that Mann heard from his wife's physician, Dr Jessen, on his brief visit to the sanatorium in Davos. Suddenly, it seems as if the mountain atmosphere is just as likely to bring out an incipient case of TB as it is to resolve an established one. Hans has a chance to show just how good a patient he can be. In the room housing the radiology apparatus he catches a glimpse of 'what he never thought it would be vouchsafed him to see: he looked into his own grave'. The none-too-solid flesh can be penetrated—'the flesh in which he walked disintegrated, annihilated, dissolved in vacant mist'—and its parts viewed as negative images quite separately from the living breathing body, and held up to the light for scrutiny. Hans has become exquisitely image-conscious, like the other patients of the Berghof who pass the time observing their 'interior portraits'. They are not disturbed by what might seem the ultimate dehumanising experience: the ghostly aseptic images of their lung-fields—cavities full of shadows—have become a kind of consolation prize for their inability to grasp the reality of their bodily affliction.

Momentous epistemological changes are just around the corner. As Bettyann Holtzmann writes in her history of medical imaging *Naked to the Bone*, the X-ray undermined not only Victorian ideas of propriety and private parts, it affected 'the self-perception of an entire culture'. On the front in 1914, radiologists worked in tandem with surgeons, using relatively primitive devices to localise bullets and shrapnel in soft tissue; and X-ray fluoroscopes entered civilian life not long afterwards, as a gimmick for fitting shoes. Since then, of course, imaging techniques have become ever more sophisticated, revealing first soft tissues, then, with the advent of ultrasound, nuclear magnetic resonance and positron emission tomography, the detailed internal structure and even metabolic activity of living tissues.

Yet which illness more visibly exposes the delusion of mistaking an image of a disease process for the true reality of the *logos* incarnate in the human form than tuberculosis—the cavitating disease? Hofrat Behrens might find the whole business of this new technology 'spooky' but he doesn't react to the X-ray films in the same way as his patients. For him, the image is a sign that can be used to uphold his physical findings or confirm advancement of the disease: it is a *demonstration*. It is metaphor-free; it lacks any imaginative 'after-image'. In the very best of cases, it ought to serve as the prelude to rational action. What his patients see in their X-rays is of a different order: for them the image-symbol is an *evocation*. It gives the old name for the disease an ironic twist: 'consumption' was thought to spiritualise the person even as it consumed the body, so that the inner glow of the soul could shine forth. It is an odd business, this idolising of X-rays...

Now that Hans can safely call the sanatorium his home, he is free to pursue his love interest. Madame Chauchat (her name is a double pun on the French word for whispering and her sexually alluring felinity) proves to be a seductive and elusive personality. To his vexation, she refuses to take his illness seriously. Settembrini, of course, detests her, seeing her as a telluric force that will disrupt the brotherhood of enlightened men. Yet the 'wicked, riotously sweet hour' Hans enjoys with her on Carnival night— seven years of hanging around a sanatorium for one hour of bliss—probes his pedestrian soul. He declares his love for her in the most stilted French (which the first English translator of Mann's novels sensibly left in the original): 'Let me take in the scent of your pores and brush the down—O human image made of water and protein, destined for the shape of the tomb: let me perish, my lips against yours!' Hans verbally lays bare his soul, in the kind of purple prose only an engineer would drum up; and then he takes possession of her soul physically, in the form of his most 'intimate' possession, the X-ray plate of her lung. Clawdia leaves the sanatorium almost immediately after their night of passion, and Hans embarks on a long course of reading and studying.

The cure for heartbreak is a curriculum.

The battle for a soul

In Clawdia's absence, Hans takes up the part of the medieval Everyman in a modern morality play. Settembrini and his new foil, Leo Naphta, a Polish Jew converted to Catholicism who has taken up lodgings in the village below the Berghof, become God and the Devil fighting it out for the young man's soul—or mouthpieces for the antithetic arguments that convulsed twentieth-century history.

Many of their sermonettes do indeed offer 'the great disputation on sickness and health' that Mann hoped for his novel. According to Settembrini, the high-toned Italian liberal and Freemason, the purpose of modern medicine is, through hygiene and social reform, to allow reason and enlightenment to triumph over all the contingencies of disease. To combat the sufferings of the flesh has a moral dimension to it, insofar as health will ultimately be identified with virtue. He reports, for instance, on the work of the League for the Organisation of Progress, the goal of which is nothing less than utopia: the total elimination of human suffering through total knowledge. 'Famous European specialists, physicians, psychologists, and economists will share in the composition of this encyclopaedia of suffering, and the general editorial bureau at Lugano will act as the reservoir to collect all the articles which shall flow into it.'

This is outright *niaiserie* to Naphta. Nothing could be more detestable than a normalised ethics for living. True spirituality and freedom are bound not to an anodyne veneration of the healthy body, but to a stoic acceptance of bodily infirmity and suffering. Being human is to be ill. 'Man was essentially ailing, his state of unhealthiness was what made him man. There were those who wanted to make him "healthy", to make him "go back to nature", when, the truth was, he never had been "natural".' Naphta, who sounds at times uncannily like a member of the Frankfurt School or even Michel Foucault, argues that the normal has always lived on 'the achievements of the abnormal'. What counts is 'iron allegiance, discipline, denial of the individual' at the service of 'the revolution of antihumane backlash'.

Naphta seems to have all the persuasive arguments, yet nothing he says ever suggests a man who means well, certainly not by young Hans Castorp, for whom his reasoning is often way above his head. Settembrini, on the other hand, is quick to notice that Naphta's thinking proceeds essentially through 'malice'.

When Clawdia returns to the sanatorium, it is in the company of her lover, Mynheer Pieter Peeperkorn, a retired colonial coffee-planter from the Netherlands. He is a gift of sorts from Clawdia Chauchat to her 'little German Hänschen', although he is hardly likely to think so at first. Peeperkorn is the fatherly but vital man whose role it is to teach Hans how to be a master of antinomies. Although Thomas Mann admitted he had modelled Peeperkorn on the German writer Gerhart Hauptmann, he seems in his embodiment of the sexual, the instinctual unconscious and the naturally religious to have stepped out of one of D. H. Lawrence's more exotic novels: the eldest character in the book is a voluptuary of stupendous personality—'though blurred'. This inarticulacy is no disadvantage. Hans is forced to admit that his soul-teachers are dwarfs beside Peeperkorn. His presence at their debates, which he mocks with a series of tics and gestures, makes their verbal skills seem trivial and unimportant. Peeperkorn's mission at the sanatorium appears to be to make Hans aware of the 'sacraments of pleasure'. He has a duty to *feel*. For brief moments, Nietzsche had written in his early work *The Birth of Tragedy*, we become 'primordial Being itself, and feel its indomitable desire for being, and joy in existence'. Even Clawdia is outshone by the bombastic enthusiasms of this primitivist, whose shock-confession to Hans is his impotence—'a cosmic catastrophe, an irreconcilable horror'. The vessel that spouts the gospel of health is cracked. To be impotent and a sexual mystic can hardly be a happy condition. And sure enough, a short time later, Peeperkorn takes his life on a picnic by a waterfall using a baroque little gadget containing poison. Soon Clawdia leaves the sanatorium for good and Hans is cast again into dudgeon.

This irruption of vitalist philosophy into the becalmed atmosphere of the Berghof is still not enough to make Hans quit the mountain. His explorations of the occult, in which he is encouraged by Behrens' assistant, the ambiguous psychoanalyst Krokowski—who is described as an 'idealist of the pathological'—bring him to another dark room and an apparition of his dead cousin Joachim dressed in a field uniform and wearing what appears to be a 'steel pot' on his head. It is a disconcerting vision which reverses the 'enlightenment' of the earlier X-ray room experience. 'Hans Castorp liked the darkness, it mitigated the queerness of the situation. And in its justification he recalled the darkness of the X-ray room, and how they had collected themselves, and "washed their eyes" in it, before they "saw".' Called up by a medium, Hans mumbles his apologies to the wraith of Joachim—who so resembled him that they had been called the 'Gemini twins'—and, in a Settembrini-like gesture, throws on the light.

Their frivolous desecration of the dead is over; and we sense that the magic of the mountain might just be starting to wear off.

An abrupt end is also in sight for the debating circle. After a general deterioration in the atmosphere at the Berghof (mirroring the conflicts in Europe that led up to the war), Settembrini and Naphta's intellectual cut-and-thrust loses its gentlemanly tone, and sinks into nasty bickering, with the former accusing the latter of infamy—of 'misleading unsettled youth'. A duel is arranged; but Settembrini casually fires his revolver into the air, refusing to shed blood, and offers his body to his rival. Naptha, enraged by Settembrini's refusal to use his weapon, shouts 'Coward!' and shoots himself through the head. Death and the daemonic turn out to have been in cahoots. It is the novel's climax—an episode entirely in the manner of that famously drastic classic German author Heinrich von Kleist—though it is hardly its resolution. The gunshot on the mountain signals the more famous one soon to ring out more than four hundred miles away in the flatlands: the Archduke Ferdinand's assassination prevents Hans from eking out his life indefinitely at the sanatorium. The first rumblings of the Great War finally enter the novel, like chairs being toppled in a drawing room. In the final, film-like epilogue to the novel, we see Hans advancing over the mists of a battlefield, bayonet in his hand, humming to himself the Schubert song 'Der Lindenbaum' (The Linden Tree) that once besotted him in the Berghof. He had first heard it on the gramophone, another kind of machine brought in to lighten the lives of the Berghof guests.

Looking down from heaven

Mann's conclusion is the most unsettling part of the novel, and not just because it falls in the shadow of the mountain of text that precedes it. His epilogue is a stilted delirium.

The first soldiers to go over the top in 1914 were the first victims of technological warfare, a horrifying inferno to be run under the guidance of the coolly functional engineer types Hans had actually trained to become. (Given his training in naval architecture, perhaps Mann ought to have placed his novice engineer in an office designing one of the advanced battleships the Germans were busily rolling down the slipways in an attempt to outdo the Royal Navy's dreadnoughts.) And there is another realisation. For over seven hundred pages we have been preoccupied with Hans Castorp's *Bildung*, his education—and what is its likely outcome? He is about to fall in the mud of a war that will not only nullify his existence but render the entire world of values that created him as archaic and irrecuperable as that of his Uncle James. The Great War certainly made it easier to die as an idealist than live like one: it was the turning point in the modern surge of cynicism about authority and superiors and people in command generally. Any writer who presumed to address warfare after 1918 would have to walk over dead bodies. Mann's touchingly rhetorical farewell to 'life's delicate child' is barely camouflage enough to prevent us from seeing that treading on corpses is precisely what they, hero and author, are both are doing in that final scene. It will also be noted that the young soldiers—those 'feverish lads'—have the same flushed face as Hans in his heightened state on the magic mountain.

In the commentary he wrote in English in 1953 for the American edition of *The Magic Mountain*, Mann observed: 'Such institutions as the Berghof were a typical pre-war phenomenon. They were only possible in a capitalistic economy that was still functioning well and normally. Only under such a system was it possible for patients to remain there year after year at the family's expense. *The Magic Mountain* became the swan song of that form of existence. Perhaps it is a general rule that epics descriptive of some particular phase of life tend to appear as it nears its end. The treatment of tuberculosis has entered upon a different phase today; and most of the Swiss sanatoria have become sports hotels.'

While it is true that the discovery of streptomycin by Albert Schatz in 1943, the first effective pharmaceutical cure for TB, led to the closure on a massive scale of spas and sanatoriums, the phenomenon of leaving the 'flatland' for what might be called recreational medical treatments actually grew considerably. In some European countries these treatments are still funded by the national health systems. As the post-war French and German governments were the first to grasp, medical tourism could be seamlessly integrated into the macroeconomics of their respective national economies. These are the naturalistic 'experiments in regeneration' that Naphta ridicules in the novel. The word Mann used to describe the heightening of Hans Castorp's personality—'*Steigerung*'—now has its primary meaning in the economic field, where it denotes increased productivity. It was, in fact, one of Goethe's key terms: intensification is what he saw as the propensity of organic phenomena to manifest themselves in ever more complex forms, to push skywards in 'a state of ever-striving ascent'. Mann had perhaps not fully anticipated how grand bourgeois families would be replaced by mass consumers with a sense of entitlement and enormous appetites, after the libidinal revolution of the 1960s, for restorative leisure. This was a key element of Herbert Marcuse's once famous notion of 'repressive tolerance', by means of which citizens are kept too busy with the delights of consumerism and demands of fashion to pay any attention to reforming society (itself a distraction from what Blaise Pascal claimed was the need to attend to the care of our immortal souls).

Under modern conditions, that delicious temporary sensation of being simultaneously above the fray, embedded in the elements (most pleasurably in the amniotic surround of a spa) or caught in a bubble of luxurious rarefaction, can be had collectively. It is not just German philosophers who get the chance to look down from heaven on the flatland far below. Now, as employees who have paid their medical insurance premiums, clients can ask their doctor to send them on a 'cure'—to a place where they can partake in an atmosphere of the most gently enforced discipline, segregation and submission to orders from above, accompanied the while by a piped Haydn or Mozart quartet.

Visiting a spa or sanatorium is the equivalent in medicine of adopting the pastoral mode in the arts.

Committed now to nothing more than our well-being, our principal guides in the art of living are doctors, not philosophers. It is Settembrini's ethics that prevail, even though the radical critique of medicine's largely humane accomplishments is pure Naphta. The contemporary German philosopher Peter Sloterdijk—who once wrote an epic novel about the beginnings of psychoanalysis called *Der Zauberbaum* (The Magic Tree)—lists in the third volume of his massive phenomenological account of modernity *Spheres*, a book with something of the grand synoptic reach of Mann's novel, the zones in our culture where we can find something of the magic mountain atmosphere: 'Even where illness does not define the very *modus vivendi*, it remains in the background as a constant possibility: fitness scenes, wellness and diet regimes, the smoothly organised and inward-looking worlds of the spa towns, the balneological retreats and the high-altitude castles for coughers would be inconceivable without it.' These are the various stations of the therapeutic good life. As an older Naphta avatar, Carl Jung, once wrote: 'the gods have become diseases'.

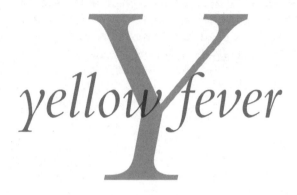

yellow fever

The Life and Times of Ernst Weiss

EXPERIMENTAL WRITING AND THE MEDICAL ORDER

1

A close literary friend of Franz Kafka, especially in the crucial period leading up to the outbreak of the Great War when Kafka famously decided not to marry his long-suffering fiancée Felice Bauer, Ernst Weiss is an almost entirely unknown figure outside German literature. Although his collected works take up sixteen volumes in the centenary German edition published in 1982 by Suhrkamp, *Georg Letham: Physician and Murderer*—resourcefully translated by Joel Rotenberg and published by the enterprising New York house Archipelago—is only the fourth of his novels to appear in English.

Born in 1882 in the Moravian city of Brünn, then a Habsburg possession (now Brno in the Czech Republic), Weiss studied medicine at the universities of Prague and Vienna where he became acquainted with many celebrated medical figures including Julius

Schnitzler and Sigmund Freud. It was a yet more famous doctor of the day who was to become Weiss' mentor: Emil Theodor Kocher, professor of surgery in Bern and winner of the Nobel Prize for Medicine in 1909 for his work on the thyroid gland. (That wasn't his only contribution to medicine: every physician who has ever worked in an emergency room has enacted Kocher's four-step manoeuvre for correcting an anterior dislocation of the humerus at the shoulder joint.) Kocher was a father-figure for Weiss, and seems to have supplied the model for the 'good doctor' depicted in so many of his novels. He many even have helped Weiss develop as a writer, since he required his assistants to write full-scale medical reports, a genre whose conventions are apparent in the writings of any physician in the early years of the last century, notably Freud himself, who commented more than once on the structural resemblances between the *Novelle* and his case histories. (Doing clinical work on the language was how many physician-writers got started in their career, but Kocher is perhaps a unique instance of the surgeon as literary lion.)

Weiss' most decisive experiences in medicine happened during his period as a ship's doctor, when he visited the Far East and Japan (although Joseph Roth once ribbed that he never went on land and 'stayed in his cabin to write'), and as a regimental doctor in the Austrian Army during the Great War. By 1921, he was living in Berlin and for all his personal prickliness, programmat-ically lurid Expressionism and partiality for characters *in extremis*, was enjoying a bit of success as a novelist and playwright. Like so many Jewish-born writers of his generation, he quit Germany after the burning of the Reichstag and returned to Prague to look after his ailing mother; after her death he headed for Paris, where he was forced to eke out a meagre existence as a translator and had to turn to better-off friends like Thomas Mann and Stefan Zweig for financial assistance.

Ernst Weiss died, of self-inflicted wounds, in the Hôpital Lari-boisière in June 1940 just hours after the Wehrmacht marched into Paris.

2

For a long time, Weiss was a name for a few rare specialists in English solely on account of the disturbing psychohistory of his last but oddly docile novel *The Eyewitness*, whose publication in the USA in 1977 had more to do with the growing field of what Mel Brooks would probably call 'Hitler studies' than any signal interest in Weiss as a literary figure.

While living in Paris, Weiss apparently met Dr Edmund Forster, a renowned neurologist who had specialised during the 1914–18 war in the new phenomenon of battlefield trauma: it was he who treated corporal Adolf Hitler in the closing months of 1918 for an episode of 'hysterical blindness' after a gas attack at Ypres. A few weeks after his visit to the émigré circles in Paris, Forster was found dead in his home at the University of Greifswald, an unlikely suicide; and Hitler's medical file disappeared from history. Five years later Weiss wrote *The Eyewitness*: it survived the war and the spoliation of his papers including the diary Weiss regarded as his masterpiece by the Gestapo after his death only because it had been submitted for a literary competition in New York (which it failed to win). In a brief scene in the novel, its medical hero indulges the unsighted Corporal 'A.H.' when the latter hysterically refuses to contemplate Germany's capitulation. The doctor puts his patient under hypnosis and suggests to him that his eyes have indeed been scarred by the mustard gas. It is a white lie to flatter his patient's vanity, and deny any psychosomatic element in his inability to see.

He tells his patient that only a truly exceptional man with 'blind faith in himself'—a romantic artist in the mould of one of the great religious leaders of the past—will have the force of personality to restore himself to sight. And his hypnotic suggestion works. Cure of his imaginary blindness opened the way for the ultimate confidence man to begin his career of spectacular ill will. *Mein Kampf* suggests a conversion experience of some kind altered Hitler's nature at the end of Germany's lost war. The clinical art had spilled over, as W. H. Auden once warned, 'from creating a world of language into the dangerous and forbidden task of trying to create a human being'.

It is easy to see why such a story of deviance and doctors appealed to Weiss. From his very first novel, *Die Galeere* ('The

Galley'), he was taken with the figure of the doctor as hero: it is not unkind to see him as writing a highbrow variety of the ever popular romantic *Arztroman* or 'doctor novel'. Although its equivalent in the English-speaking world (now largely superseded by TV series) has acquainted us with the idea that even priestly 'demigods in white' can be fallible, Weiss' figures are deeply implicated in far more serious and morally dubious business than silly pranks and affairs with nurses. There is a largely unspoken assumption in his work that those who fake the virtues are especially dangerous in a modern technological society. His character 'A.H.', for instance, is an incorrigible fantasiser, but he is not exactly a liar: it would be more accurate to say that his whole life is one gigantic lie in which there is no absolute except the truth of his imagination. Much in the same way, the not entirely reliable first-person narrator in *Georg Letham: Physician and Murderer*—first published in 1931 by Paul Zsolnay Verlag in Vienna—declares in the foreword to the novel: 'The profound, truly disastrous disorder and futility of nature and the world—what in the scientific realm we call the pathological, in the moral realm the criminal—these are constant'.

That is the preamble of a convicted murderer. Letham is a reverse Hamlet: he is out to avenge not his father's unlawful death but his father's killing of his own soul. Weiss is an early explorer of the inward turn that has made 'trauma' a contemporary psychological concept in which perceived cause and manifest effect are difficult to tell apart. The first third of the novel is taken up with events leading up to the murder of his almost twenty-year-older, wealthier wife, whose devotion to him has been 'doglike'. Self-important in his devotion to science, Letham seems to move effortlessly from research to his lucrative private practice as surgeon and gynaecologist. (His person conjures up the glamorous society doctor depicted in trenchcoat, the one hand on his microscope and the other holding a test-tube, in Tamara de Lempicka's 1929 painting *Portrait of Doctor Boucard*.) 'Illnesses interested me, the ill did not', Letham confesses, drawing attention to the dissevering of reason and emotion that marks his entire life. He is seeking an *ex post facto* rationale for his crime, as if it had been a dispassionate intellectual act, when what he says suggests he had often fantasised about it. Indeed, it happens almost nonchalantly one evening when she 'asks for it': mistaking a vial lying in his study for morphine, his wife begs him to administer some pain relief. What he injects is 'Toxin Y', a deadly product of his own research.

Arrogant about his motives ('Ultimately only I could judge this crime') and seemingly indifferent to his fate, Letham is sentenced to hard labour at C., an unspecified penal colony in Central America. It is a Devil's Island, where the locals live in terror of coming down with yellow fever ('Y.F.'). As in Thomas Mann's TB-haunted mountain top, a microbial illness threatens an islanded society with dissolution. Little by little, Letham's mortuary precision begins to buckle under the strain of real anguish. The young man, March, with whom he is quartered falls in love with him; and although Letham is clearly fascinated by March he is unable to return his affection. It is only when he himself develops feelings for a young Portuguese girl entrusted to his care and whose life he is unable to save that he, for the first time, feels something like emotion. The veneer of objectivity is showing cracks.

A penal colony has to rely on people with skills, even when they are convicted murderers: Letham is doctoring again. The subsequent saga of research and discovery is clearly based on the pioneering—and successful—attempts to eradicate 'Y.F.' from Havana in the 1890s and William Reed's proving of the 'mosquito hypothesis' during the American building of the Panama canal in the 1900s (the French had had to abandon an earlier attempt at construction in the 1880s because of the exceptionally high mortality rate among workers and engineers as a result of malaria and yellow fever): Letham discovers a sense of professional purpose in researching the epidemic's origins.

'Scientific work is a joy' he confesses; he has even 'become fond of life'. Like many pioneering researchers, he and his colleagues allow themselves to be infected in order to determine whether their specially bred mosquitoes are indeed vectors for Y.F. But the experimenter in him—'The experimenter is like God, but on a small scale'—gets the better of this moment of self-sacrifice, when he fails to intervene on catching sight of an escaped mosquito, in all likelihood infected, poised on the nape of his colleague's pregnant wife. He wants to see whether the infection will be transmitted to the child *in utero*. It is the beginning of the end of his relationship with March, who spots this act of dereliction.

Although Letham and his colleagues are successful in eradicating the blight—'We gradually cleaned up an area larger than Europe'—the sentence that concludes the book is emotionally telling: 'I disappeared into the crowd, and that is for the best.' Dr Letham has the measure of himself at last.

3

The New York publisher Archipelago is to be congratulated on commissioning and publishing the translation of this long novel. It is a pity nobody could be found to provide it with an introduction, though, or even a few notes about its medical background. Weiss' own life is sufficiently if undeservingly obscure as to require as much context as it can get, and the natural history of the disease that punctuates the course of the novel is not entirely as Weiss presents it: he appears to have confused the mode of transmission of yellow fever, a haemorrhagic viral illness vectored by female mosquitoes of the genus *Aedes aegypti* (in those days, and in the novel, called *Stegomyia fasciata*), with leptospirosis, a bacterial disease of the liver contracted through contact with infected mammalian urine. It used to be known as 'rat catcher's yellows', and was common in the trenches in the Great War. Its fulminant form is known as Weil's disease.

Kafka's reservations about Weiss' editorial talents were not ill-founded either: the entire first third of the novel (leading up to the murder of Letham's wife) ought to have been presented as a short flashback. The whole thing creaks under the weight of its symbolic superstructure: Thomas Mann might have imposed a complex 'rule of sevens' on the realism of *The Magic Mountain*, but the outcome there was rather more convincing and sustained by Mann's understated humour. The very Kafkaesque obsession with all-conquering fathers—Georg Letham senior is a Polar explorer as well as a rat-exterminator—raises more questions than it answers, too. Hamlet's actual contribution to events is perhaps most felt in his advice in the original play to his mother, Queen Gertrude: 'Assume a virtue if you have it not.' Assuming virtues is plainly a perilous invitation in an inverted moral order. If Kafka, in some of his short stories, provided the imaginative backdrop to the geography of Nazi horror, Ernst Weiss seems to have had an ominous sense that monstrous programmes might descend on society through the workings of people able to assume a mask of goodness even as they pursue a radical evil. Hitler, certainly, was always very keen on medical metaphors; and his political method for resolving complex social problems was all too often that of biological expediency.

In a novel that explores the ethics of experimental science, the more fitting character to adopt from Shakespeare would have been Iago, not Hamlet. He is the true exponent of Francis Bacon's contemporaneous idea of putting nature on the rack. Letham murders his wife not because his father has bungled the job of bringing him up but because she is the one person who knows him—knows him in the intimate Biblical sense, since his disgust with her is closely linked to his compulsion to abuse her sexually: their relationship, as he acknowledges, is sado-masochistic. The fact that he refuses other people this mutuality of knowledge is significant. He is after scientific knowledge in Bacon's classic sense, to stand *over* what he is investigating, which is a stance nobody can adopt in an authentically human relationship.

In Shakespeare's play, Iago utters his coldly dismissive final comment, 'What you know, you know', only when he has reduced Othello to a thing. His understanding of other people's desires (and how to manipulate them) is Machiavellian in its subtlety but he gives no sign of understanding his own reasons for doing what he does, a phenomenon that is entirely consistent with a self that relates to others only negatively. Indeed, the recognition that he is parasitic on the creation he despises—'I am nothing if not critical'—shifts an otherwise empty soliloquy into the vertigo of infinite regress.

There are, however, a couple of expressionistic nightmare scenes in *Georg Letham* which attest to Weiss' talent for what is recognisably a filmic style: a lab dog with part of its cranium removed and electrodes still implanted in its grey matter escapes its cage and scampers, barking with excitement, into the medical amphitheatre, only to have the remaining brains knocked out of it in a *coup de grâce* administered by the admired student who eventually becomes Letham's colleague in C.; and a typhus corpse buried at sea fails to sink, gradually unwinds from its grave-sheet, and is tossed 'in mad high spirits' by the dolphins cavorting in the wake of the ship.

Both these scenes bring on animals: the entire novel is haunted by creatures surviving—and even thriving—on the boundaries of human society. First the rats that dart in and out of Letham's narrative, from his father's 'Rat Palace' to the scenes of his own nastiness; then the mosquitoes, which decimate the population of C. and cut a strip off human ambition; and finally the viruses that are the hidden but effective cause of Y.F. Outsiders all, but only Georg Letham presumes to set himself up as a critic.

Ultimately the novel itself is a kind of experiment: just how far can we trust such an unreliable narrator? Weiss knows we can't entirely condemn his repulsive experimenter: our culture long ago endorsed the notion that the right to know is absolute and overriding. Knowledge of what preys on us is one thing; the truth of the matter, eroded by those disruptive rats, is always going to be something else.

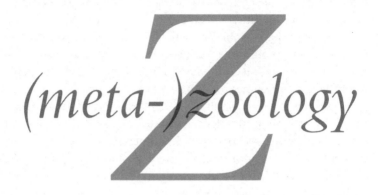

Parasites

OR, HOW TO FLYPE A METAPHOR

PARASITE: *An organism that for some or all of its lives, lives on or in the body or cell of another organisms (host), deriving its food from the host. The host does not benefit from the association and is often harmed by it. Human parasites include viruses, bacteria, protozoons and worms.*
— Cambridge Encyclopedia of Evolution

PITY: *A squandering of feeling, a parasite harmful to moral health.*
— Friedrich Nietzsche

FLYPE: *v.t. Chiefly Scottish. 1. Strip off (the skin, etc.), peel, flay. 2. Turn up or down, fold back; turn inside out.*
— Shorter Oxford English Dictionary

Lifted out of their hiding places parasites may look strange and monstrous, but only as strange and monstrous as organisms which, to gain their ends, are resolved to one nervous or narrow form of themselves: dependency is organised in such a way as to seem almost a virtue. The host is substance and nutriment; its inner dark is burrowed into and fed on; the parasite thrives and grows; and what results is a spectacular triumph existing solely by means of its attachment. A parasite is all in its feeding. In fact, it is in the nature of things that this very attachment offers the host a means of protection against the parasite. Soon the host is innocently whistling again, happy in the conviction that the microworld of parasites he can't see coincides in every detail with the macroworld made squeaky clean by such essential gadgets as bars of soap, vacuum cleaners and wet-wipes.

Parasites exist, it would seem, despite water purification, sewage disposal, free school milk, and medicine itself. Even, it would seem, despite Engel's description of the Manchester slums in 1844, where Manchester now yields to cities like Lagos, Bombay, Nairobi or Lima. Adolf Hitler, another world-reformer, was fond of the word he correctly recognised as social Darwinism's gift to *amour propre*; unfortunately nobody ever bothered to read his turgid ideas about what-to-do-with-those-who-sup-at-the-tables-of-others, written down in black and white; which is why we ended up with the twentieth century. And the twentieth century, as we know, was just a coda to the marvellous nineteenth, which thought the future would work out just the way humans wanted it to: the overwhelming success of Pasteur's germ theory turned—and certainly not just in the scientific imagination—all talk about health and illness into a vision of armed camps and invasions, with hygiene as a pre-emptive strike against enemy forces. It's not surprising, a hundred years later, that epidemiology (coined as a word in 1873, and meaningful as a science only after the Second World War) looks like catastrophe theory in slow motion.

We should examine some examples of what we're talking about. Take malaria, for instance. It means 'bad air' in Italian, is the paludal or marsh disease in French, and has proved to be a disease of great resourcefulness notwithstanding the rather complicated nature of the sexual life of the organism *Plasmodium*, which was first written up by Sir Ronald Ross and his less feted Indian assistant, Muhammad Bux. The sexual life of *Plasmodium*, which in zoological terms is a protozoon (single-celled creature), takes place in the salivary gland of the *Anopheles* mosquito; the other part of its life cycle requires colonisation of liver cells in a specific mammalian species. Infection occurs when the mosquito puts its mouthpart, which is a small but effective hypodermic syringe, into your integument and sucks without obvious display of table manners at the puncture site. Mosquito saliva, of course, is where *Plasmodium* tends to hang about. Once the host is inoculated, liver cells are used for a while as incubators until they rupture, perhaps—as I used to imagine when I studied tropical medicine in London a decade ago—under the shock of being defined by the bristly word 'schizont', sending thousands of invading, and equally bristly merozoites (the first asexual stage) into the circulation. There they go out like preachers and settle in naive young red cells, develop into female or male sexual cells, and wait for an obliging second mosquito to come and airlift them from the scene of their successful coup. This red cell stage causes the periodic fever that comes with malaria, and each species (there are four in humans) has its own pattern of febrile paroxysm. The prime method of diagnosing malaria hasn't changed since the salad days of empire, and relies on microscopic identification of the *Plasmodium* parasites in thick and thin blood films. Recent attempts to develop simple dipstick serological assays have run into problems of either cost or lack of specificity, although one method based on a soluble protein antigen of *P. falciparum* was able to detect evidence of infection in a four-thousand-year-old Egyptian mummy. Moreover, hopes of a vaccine against *P. falciparum*, such as the SPf66 synthetic peptide which incorporates various merozoite proteins and was tested recently in children in Columbia, keep running up against evolutionary paradigms; namely, the capacity of the protozoon to modify its internal proteins through natural selection quicker than we can invent ways of stopping those proteins from getting fresh with blood cells. In tacit recognition of which, a sequence tag map of the *P. falciparum* genome is now being constructed so that potential targets for drugs and vaccines can be identified.

One version of the evolutionary paradigm runs like this: once humans migrated from the savannah to moist places where they could do their laundry and drink water out of old tin cans, and *Plasmodium* reached an understanding with its host in terms of population infection rates, an amazing number of people turned up at the local Happy Africa Family clinic with its corrugated tin facade and undressed concrete walls and were found to have evidence of sickle cell disease and foetal haemoglobin in their veins. Sickle cell disease isn't that common generally, but hete-rozygotes—people with one copy of a normal haemoglobin gene and one copy of an abnormal sickle-cell gene—can be found in their thousands in West Africa. Selection in the human population retains the abnormal gene since it prevents the parasite gaining ready admission to the red cells. On the other hand, natural selec-tion, being entirely indiscriminate as far as genetic base-pairs go, works on the parasite populations too: chloroquine resistance was first reported in South America in 1961 and has since been observed in nearly all endemic areas. Vaccines aren't likely to be more successful, unless they can anticipate new antigenic config-urations before they happen. Any talk of eradicating malaria is, in the long view of the evolutionist, a pipe-dream: such gorgeously coloured bubbles might have blown from Geneva not so many years ago, but enough to give the impression that an epoch has lapsed in terms of optimism. In 1995, 2.1 million people died of malaria across the world.

Once, and not so long ago, parasitology itself seemed to exist only as a vector for the export of optimism to the Third World. Nowa-days, tropical medicine books are more correctly called manuals to the diseases of warm climates, since it would be an error (and one I have fostered entirely to my own ends in this essay) to suppose that the effects of disease are due solely to parasites: poverty is the most important risk factor for morbidity around the equatorial belt, and is likely to become even more so in this century. Parasitism itself is a condition of the rural poor, not of city-dwellers, which is why people in the know (like epidemiologists) refer on the one hand to the now largely defunct discipline of tropical medicine, which was an invention of British, French and Belgian colonial policy at the end of the nineteenth century, notably the period of Joseph Chamberlain's stewardship of the colonies, *and* to medicine in the tropics. In fact, the fastest growing diseases in the tropics these days are commonplace 'western' conditions: hypertension, ischaemic heart disease and non-insulin-dependent diabetes.

Whatever the claim these three diseases have on our attention, and most doctors know them like the back of their hand, malaria is a good example of evolution in action, and shows why the word 'natural' in natural selection sometimes seems a bit forced. This is the first quality of parasites to be held against them: their ability to hitch rides and squeeze through loopholes and generally take credit for being hangers-on; in short, their opportunism. The very dynamism of evolution seems to depend on sameness at one remove from itself.

Anopheline mosquitoes also transmit filiariasis, which is an infection caused by long slender worms. *Wuchereria bancrofti* is one family of these filarial worms: they tend to be about 4–6 cm long, home in on the tubes and ductules of the human lymphatic system, and can live there quite snugly for a decade or two. In a mild infection, it's possible for male and female to spend the rest of their life unsuccessfully trying to find each other in the body's sluice pipes and sumps and end up not producing any baby worms at all. Unlike their parents, immature worms (microfilariae) prefer the small blood vessels of the lungs where they hole up during the day and emerge into the general circulation at night, with rush hour between 10 at night and 2 in the morning, in the hope that a visiting mosquito might vacuum them in with the rest of its blood-meal. (As with malaria, the female anopheline mosquito may of course deposit the infective larvae while feeding.) That this tidal phenomenon should occur at all is remarkable, since it posits an ability on the part of the filariae to read the human host's circadian clock while banking on the regularity of female mosquitoes. In fact, there are two periodic forms of *W. bancrofti*: one which comes out at night, the nocturnally periodic form, and is transmitted by night-biting mosquitoes; the other a diurnally subperiodic form, which is transmitted by *Aedes* mosquitoes in the Pacific that prefer to bite by day. Since infected people living in the Nicobar Islands in the bay of Bengal have daytime tidal infections in a region where they should have nighttime (the nocturnal form is prevalent in most of Asia), ethnologists have hypothesised that their great-grandparents originally migrated westwards across the sea from south-east Asia, not long enough ago though for natural selection to have reset the worm clocks. Or for the disease to have died out in the Nicobar Islands for that matter.

In filariasis, it's usually the body's urge to show off its immunological arsenal which causes symptoms of disease, rather than worms lurking about in the recesses of the lungs or lymphatics.

Often the only index of parasitic infection (of any parasitic infection) is a high count of some specialised white blood cells called eosinophils. Eosinophils are part of the cell-mediated response; they contain granules of toxic proteins and chemicals and regulate other defence cells. At a local level, cell-mediated response is rapidly followed by antibody production in the upstream lymphatic ducts. If this kind of immunological war gets under way, neither side really wins: the lymphatic system clogs up with scar tissue, calcified worm parts and a jungle of obliterating fibrosis—and the outside landscape changes. Lymphoedema may follow the initial attack on the lymphatics: deposition of collagen and secondary infection gives rise to the infamous swelling condition known as elephantiasis. This used to compel unfortunate older gentlemen in the South Seas to transport their varicose testicles down to market in a wheelbarrow while hoping that nobody would mistake them for a pawpaw.

This is the second quality of parasites: their periodicity; that is, their ability to rebound on us like inherited and derivative modes of thinking.

Guinea worm (*Dracunculus medinensis*) is another, more spectacular parasitic worm, transmitted in larval form by a fresh-water crustacean called *Cyclops*. *Dracunculus* is big enough to see. In fact, the adult female is as big as a knitting needle. It occurs mainly in the rain forests and swamp areas of West Africa, and lives by vagabonding around the body's connective tissues. After mating, the male is absorbed by the female. Unlucky patients sometimes catch sight of one crossing the tissues beneath the skin without so much as a by-your-leave, but generally the adult females draw attention to themselves only once their uterus gets bulky. At this point they become geotropic, that is they make a break for Mother Earth by the shortest possible route. That means if *Dracunculus* is in the abdominal tissues it heads for the genitals, if in the arms the fingers, and so on. Usually it pokes out just behind the ankle. Since the host has just woken up with a bleb on his skin where he didn't have one before, he not unnaturally tries to soothe his sore foot by bathing it in water. Whereupon the worm's head emerges, sticks out a clear tube (its uterus, where nobody but an entomologist would expect it) and discharges a cloudy jism into the water. The guinea worm is packed with some three million embryos, and even a sniff of water is enough to cause its gravid uterus to contract peristaltically, thereby expelling the huge genetic load in a few moments. Once in the water, the larvae get siphoned in by *Cyclops* and moult in its body cavity. Man drinks water, and the cycle begins anew. The Scottish poet Hugh MacDiarmid found this parasitic simile so appealing he instanced the guinea worm's uterine prolapse in his late poem *To a Friend and Fellow-Poet* as an odd naturalistic trope for his own repeated acts of cultural kamikaze:

> Is it not precisely thus we poets deliver our store,
> Our whole being the instrument of our suicidal art,
> And by the skin of our teeth 'flype' ourselves into fame?

Life goes on though, at least in West Africa, as if unpleasant things like guinea worms were merely a minor irritation: the traditional method of removing one from the view of fascinated relatives is to wrap its head around a matchstick and wind it a bit more every day until the whole worm is out. It sounds a bit like removing a shoelace which has embedded itself inadvertently in your foot, except that the people it affects hardly ever wear shoes and if they did, most likely wouldn't need to remove worms from their feet. I used to think the medical emblem of a snake coiled around Asclepius' staff (*two* snakes around Hermes' peace-restoring caduceus) was a tribute to the ability of snakes to regenerate their skin (and, by analogy, of medicine to heal the sick); it may simply be a very stylised guinea worm or two twisted around a splinter of balsa wood.

That is the third quality of parasites, and the one we recoil from with the most baroque shudder of all: their lack of scruple in taking advantage of human nature. No matter how outlandish (and it seems the freakier the better) they worm their way into our most hallowed institutions and freshly scrubbed ideas; and I haven't even mentioned the figurative possibilities of linguistic contagions like bilharzia, cestodes, jiggers and liver rot.

Clearly the systems relations of the parasitologist are far from politically neutral. Parasites need people, but what do people gain from parasites, the one-sided definition of the *Cambridge Encyclopedia of Evolution* notwithstanding? A flyped metaphor, I suppose, is the answer; a word safely anchored in literal truth that spills out into the illimitable. Yet metaphors can vitiate what they sustain. It is surprising that a philosopher as sensitive to language as Nietzsche would come up with the suggestion that 'no thinker hitherto has had the courage to measure the health of a society or of individuals by the number of parasites they can withstand' (*Daybreak*), as if such a compromising metaphor could serve as any kind of measure of public or individual 'health'. But he did; and to those of us sensitised to biological metaphors, the twentieth century seems like a long catalogue of terrible linguistic category errors, with one unscrupulous demagogue after another finding there is no limit to what can done with a vocabulary that takes its orders from Nature. Being at the bottom of the pile, 'parasite' is the hierarchical order term par excellence. In the hunt for affinities in a world where solid things keep melting into air, parasites reveal how irresistibly reflexivity colonizes not just our bodies and the production chain, but even our language. 'Only parasites tremble / On the edge of the future', wrote the Russian poet Osip Mandelstam in his 1923 poem 'My Era'. And so it proved: 'parasites' was the term favoured by the Soviet tribunals to stigmatise poets, especially when they sentenced them to hard labour.

Clearly parasites provide fantastically contrived mechanisms for avoiding the obvious, methods of burrowing deep into the architecture of human reasoning and laying blisters of dissent inside the body politic, there to trigger new ways of fear and loathing. Miroslav Holub, the Czech immunologist-poet, has this menacing close to his poem 'Parasite': 'for years the eruption will die away / and little spores of imbecile agreement / will bore into granite and wait there / like wet dynamite.' In essence, the word 'parasite' is itself metonymic for everything we don't like about everybody else. And, as a corollary, of reinforcing just how sure we are about the inestimable advantage of being ourselves. Of being *proper*. Just think about it: within ten hours of being born and deposited on the planet, pioneering streptococci have colonised babies' mouths, soon to be followed by enterococci, actinomycetes, candida, lactobacilli and other ecological golddiggers. That's what happens when children can't keep their mouths shut. Indeed that's what happens in general to human beings, who can't stop speaking in the same place where they eat—not my words, not yours, but everybody's. Then again, as that now deeply unfashionable poet Brecht once noticed in his poem 'On Thinking about Hell', the fear of being thrown on the street wears down the owners of villas no less than the denizens of shanty towns. Having guests, being hospitable and convivial, showing concern for others' welfare: these were the first linguistic codes of the human community, a first recognition that we—creatures of the natural world—love and hate in a symbolic one.

In reality, we are extravagant hosts. While writing this piece I was drawn up short to find out (as a response to Nietzsche's rhetorical challenge) just how laden we are: the average adult human is composed of about 10^{14} cells, only ten percent of which are 'human'. All nucleated cells, which accounts for a good deal of our substantial being, are basically colonies of symbiotic bacteria. And not only that, but we share most of our DNA with almost everything in the universe, including fungi and yeasts. That makes us nothing short of travelling zoos. How much courage does it take to be a zoo? We'll never know. But let me seed a virtual parasite myself: thinking we can live closer to Nature by following the Victorian creed of applied Darwinism or even imaging we can get by without greeting the neighbours has a price: exclude the symbolic, and you get its dread extruded form, the *diabolectic*.

Endnotes

A Taste of Bitter Almonds
[*British Journal of General Practice*, 2010]
Joseph Joubert's remark that 'those who have kept their personality are always enchanted by that of other people, even if in opposition to their own' might almost have been intended for Stendhal. Stendhal preserved himself by being witty. But he didn't acquire wit until he was middle-aged, at about the same time as he—a provincial and Italophile—started to esteem Paris. 'That way of improvising with a tranquil mind only came to me in 1827', he confesses.

The Plastinator
[*London Review of Books*, 2000]
Given Professor Günther (von) Hagens' partiality for pastiche, it is just as well he hasn't come across the parallel scenes in Curzio Malaparte's war novel *The Skin* (1949), in which two men are rolled over by tanks, one a persecuted Jew in the Ukraine, the other an Italian celebrating the arrival of American forces in Rome. All that is left of them is 'a skin in the shape of a man', which in the latter case is waved by colleagues as a flag.

I was gratified to see that my argument against Hagens' spurious defence of his showmanship as a 'democratisation' of anatomy received unrelated support in Susan Mattern's recent life of Galen *The Prince of Medicine* (2013). 'Anatomy is a cumulative science', she writes. 'One cannot simply cut up a corpse and find meaning in its inner structures without knowing what to look for.' Incidentally, Austin Gresham, forensic histopathologist and author of the *Colour Atlas of Forensic Pathology* (1975), was not impressed that his manual 'of every conceivable way to get to the mortuary', as the artist Mat Collishaw has described it, inspired some of the more controversial exhibits of the Britart pack, including Collishaw's own 'Bullet Hole' and Damien Hirst's notorious shark in formaldehyde. He believed the dead should be treated with that old-time concept, dignity.

It is curious that this year the first public dissections in the United Kingdom resumed after a period of 170 years (for the sum of £100 members of the public can attend a series of dissection workshops run by the University of Edinburgh to 'see under the skin and gain an understanding of how [their] body works'), even as many medical students now learn what they know about body structure from computer simulations that spare them gross anatomy's rite of passage.

Knock! Knock!
[*Medical Humanities*, 2002]
Jules Romains' play *Knock ou Le Triomphe de la Médecine* (1924) is taught in French schools, and generally very well known in its country of origin. I had the crazy idea fifteen years ago of translating the play and offering it to the BBC (or anyone else who might take it) in the hope that the film, which stars the consummate Louis Jouvet, might be broadcast in the original French with my script doing service as subtitles; and if not nationwide, then as an ethics primer for medical students. Unfortunately I was unable to interest anyone in the script, in spite of its obvious relevance in an era of 'more medicine can only be better medicine', and the manuscript is slowly yellowing in a drawer somewhere.

In a rather overheated commentary on the play in his memoir *Témoignages sur le théâtre* (1952), Jouvet uses the term 'idée-force', which I take to be a French import from German phenomenology ('Zweckidee'): I have accordingly translated it as 'guiding concept'. The Coué method namechecked in the essay was very popular in the United States for a time, being mentioned by Ferdinand, in Céline's classic novel *Voyage au bout de la nuit* (1922) when the American girl Lola accuses him of 'doing harm' by telling her that her mother's liver cancer is incurable: 'In her despair I sniffed vestiges of the Coué method.' Even then in the New World, all news had to be good news.

A Conspiracy of Good Intentions
[*British Journal of General Practice*, 2005]
The alleged partiality of ethicists has been further explored by Carl Elliott in his book *White Coat, Black Hat: Adventures on the Dark Side of Medicine* (2010) and David Healy in *Pharmageddon* (2013), which detail just how completely medicine has been absorbed into the 'health care' priorities of large-scale enterprise. Many bioethicists work now as paid consultants to pharmaceutical companies,

just as half of all anthropology graduates find jobs in industry.

What is sinister about the extraordinary (empathic) explosion of 'depression' as a diagnostic category is that it has become a basket diagnosis for the demoralisation that consumer society brings, inevitably, in its wake. In the pharmaceutical paradigm which now prevails, patients are obliged to take, sometimes for years, the antidepressants which doctors, beholden to their employer (i.e. the government), are compelled by their checklists and protocols to prescribe. Only economists will ever be able to make productive sense of it.

Insomnia (in the Bed of Being)
[*PN Review*, 2013]
'The greatest thing one man can do for another,' wrote Kierkegaard, 'insofar as each individual has to deal only with himself, is to leave him disquieted.' To be insomniac is to be haunted by thoughts that won't settle, and everything suggests that this has been the common fate of mortals since what the French call 'la nuit des temps'—when Being was anything but tucked up cosily in bed. To suffer insomnia is to experience the body as a complete stranger who refuses obstinately to do our bidding. Indeed, insomnia may be another expression for the wound that doesn't close, as in Kafka's unsettling story about the country doctor ('Uncle Siegfried').

An American Book of the Dead
[*PN Review*, 1997, as 'Man in Black, a review of Thomas Lynch's memoir *The Undertaking: Life Studies from the Dismal Trade*']
I almost surprised myself at the amount of sympathy I was able to muster for Thomas Lynch, running his father's funeral home in order to make ends meet. But then I was running a medical practice in Strasbourg strictly as a business at the time, with none of the financial cushion provided by the NHS: the issue of asking for payment directly from patients, whether suffering or not, was a challenge for me in ways I hadn't expected. Some of the predicaments aired in Lynch's book received even more emphatic treatment in the long-running HBO television drama *Six Feet Under*, which follows events in an entire family of undertakers in Los Angeles over five years. It is often rated as one of the best TV

series ever. Its creator Alan Ball attests: 'the books I found most helpful were *The Undertaking: Life Studies from the Dismal Trade* and *Bodies in Motion and at Rest: On Metaphor and Mortality*, both by Thomas Lynch, a funeral director and poet, and a brilliant, soulful writer'.

Crise de Foie
[*Süddeutsche Zeitung*, 2000, as 'Der majestätische Rang der Leber: die Franzosen und ihre Crise de Foie']
The prominence of the liver in French medicine dates to the premodern period, and the battle waged by the dogmatic Galenist and ultraconservative member of the Paris faculty Jean Riolan the Younger (1580–1657) against William Harvey's new doctrine of the circulation, which he correctly saw as questioning not only the pre-eminence of the liver as the blood-making organ but also fatally undermining the authority of his faculty and Galenic therapeutics in general. If the same blood was circulating indifferently throughout the body why should novice-doctors have to learn bleeding points? Why bleed patients at all? It was Descartes, an amateur dissector, who really saw the point of Harvey's new doctrine and enlisted it for his groundbreaking *Discours sur la méthode* (1637).

Some of the issues around 'mal de foie' are explained in Colette Mechin, 'Le foie, organe tropique dans la société traditionnelle française', in the book *Usage culturels du corps* (1997). The (notorious) reference about what to do after the orgy is from Jean Baudrillard's *La Transparence du Mal* (1990). Even Karl Marx recognised the effects of liverishness on his writing style, explaining in a letter of 1858 to his publisher Ferdinand Lassalle that his difficulty in delivering the final manuscript of his thesis on capital was due to efforts to ensure that 'the thing shouldn't be disfigured by the kind of heavy, wooden style proper to a disordered liver…'

The Moral Life of Happiness
[*Quadrant*, 2005, as 'The Homeostatics of Happiness, a review of Ziyad Marar's *The Happiness Paradox* and Carl Elliott's *Better than Well*']
Flaubert had a withering aside about the nineteenth-century search for happiness: 'To be stupid, egoistic and in good health,

those are the three conditions required in order to be happy. But if you lack the first everything is lost.' There have been scores of books since the turn of the millennium about the nature of happiness (and how to attain it); even governments haven't shied away from adopting it as an aspect of policy. Surely one of the wiser things written about the fabled state came from John Stuart Mill in 1873: 'those only are happy (I thought) who have their minds fixed on some object other than their own happiness. Aiming thus at something else they find happiness along the way.' It is adventitious. I can even remember people who used to be happy helping others. And perhaps the truth is simpler and shier still: happiness abhors analysis.

An Empty Plot
[*London Review of Books*, 2001, as 'Then It's Your Whole Life, an essay-review of Emmanuel Carrère's novel *The Adversary*']
In his various novels, Emmanuel Carrère has explored the condition of what he calls 'Uchronie'—a neologism that clearly derives from the concept of utopia. In English, this 'time out of mind' is better known in its different guises as the counterfactual novel or the 'what if' retelling of alternative history. Carrère teeters on the edge of an abyss, playing the analyst's role of non-person to perfection, but sometimes forgetting that his subject is himself a non-person: a man who turns himself into a moral paragon, lies about himself exorbitantly for eighteen years, and then murders his extended family when the truth emerges (as it was bound to do). This story gripped me when I read it, because I could see how the border situation in which I was living lent itself to this kind of moral duplicity, and raised troubling questions about the self-determining modern individual, the egoism that has no self behind it. Romand's 'integrity' is that of an empty husk.

Chekhov Goes to Sakhalin
[*British Journal of General Practice*, 2001, as 'Pages Blank as Tundra, a contribution to a special issue on deprivation in health care']
The motives for Chekhov's journey to Sakhalin are still something of a mystery. Perhaps it was, as the French might say, an 'antipsychanalyse'—James Joyce suggested in *Ulysses* that some people would rather slog it to the ends of the earth than peer

inwards. For a writer as insightful and articulate as Chekhov his 'fugue' eastwards was surely propelled less by any scepticism about the introspected self than his interest in the variety of the world: conditions in a penal colony were as worthy of note as a cherry orchard on the outskirts of Moscow. The trip to Sakhalin is an almost luridly dramatic insert in the life of a chronically unwell writer who introduced a note of sophisticated inconclusiveness and indirection into literature that is present everywhere today.

My quotes are from the excellent translation of Chekhov's report by Brian Reeve, which was published by a small press in Cambridge in 1993; an alterative (American) version is also in existence. I also relied on Donald Rayfield's classic biography (1997) and Janet Malcolm's insightful *Reading Chekhov: A Critical Journey* (2001).

Uncle Siegfried
[*Medical Humanities*, 2000]
'Where is the doctor? I'm searching the letter without reading it just to find the doctor. Where is he?' That was Kafka, writing in one of his insistent letters to Milena Jesenská during their brief if intense relationship. If 'cherchez la femme' was the motive introduced into French fiction by Alexandre Dumas, suggesting that the reason for a man's inexplicable actions was that he is either trying to cover up an affair or curry favour with a woman, then Kafka's bright idea might be said to be 'den Arzt suchen'. Kafka had little faith in what the Germans call 'school medicine' and its obsession with 'monocausal' explanations (still a prominent feature of contemporary evidence-based medicine), and he was especially impatient with doctors—and he consulted a lot of them in his relatively short life—who contradicted each other. On the other hand he showed great respect for one or two figures, including his friend Robert Klopstock, whom he called a 'born doctor' and who supported him in his final illness.

Is There Life on Earth?
[*Parnassus*, 1998]
ICD-10 is the 10th revision of the International Statistical Classification of Diseases and Related Health Problems, a coding register set up by the World Health Organization, which contains

almost 14,500 codes for signs, symptoms, findings, complaints, social circumstances, and external causes of injury or diseases. I have translated discharge letters (from the German) where doctors, rather than supply diagnoses, simply list ICD codes, a procedure that disturbed me when I first encountered it. Standardisation is an important aspect of modernity, but in this case it seemed doctors were actually conniving to reorganise the profession under a rationality that has little to do with the uncertainties that dominate the doctor-patient encounter and more with output, productivity and medicine-as-industry. The pressure to do this of course comes from the paymaster, in this case Germany's statutory health insurance funds.

This came home with even more force when my wife, who worked for a while as a district nurse in the Ortenau region of Baden told me about her rounds: in her car she carried a folder that held about a dozen laminates with bar-codes at the bottom of each page. After every visit to a patient, she had to key in the patient's details and relay information to a central databank about the nursing tasks she had just performed by scanning the applicable bar-code with a hand-held scanner. On the last page was a stand-alone code titled 'Menschliches Handeln'—a rough translation of which might be 'humane acts'. This was meant to cover time spent with the patient that couldn't be accounted for as a nursing procedure: asking patients about the weather or their grandchildren, for instance, or merely how they were feeling. It was limited to ten minutes.

Tell Me about Teeth
[unpublished, 2015]
In the same week as writing this, I read about poorer British people performing 'DIY dentistry' with kits available on the high street because of their inability to afford dental care, while cosmetic dentistry registered a record turnover in 2014 of almost one billion pounds sterling, suggesting that parts of the UK may be moving towards neo-Victorian conditions of dental distress while other parts embrace the American fixation on perfect teeth.

I ought, besides, to admit a trifle guiltily that the acclaimed contemporary novel *The Yacoubian Building* was written by the Egyptian dentist Alaa El Aswany, and had I tried harder would surely have come across other writers who happen to earn their living as dentists. Indeed, dentist-writers might be able to provide a few lessons in modesty for doctor-writers all too ready to vaunt themselves as paragons of all the virtues.

Hygiene of the Soul
[*Quadrant*, 2012]
In view of what Brecht said about the smelliness of *homo sapiens*, it is noteworthy that when his reputation was 'assassinated', thirty years after his death, in a book that detailed his covert homosexuality, exploitation of women (some of whom were supposed to have written his plays), love of money and political shiftiness, the killer stroke was delivered by those who remember him as being a particularly smelly man, an impression no doubt intensified by those cheap *krumme Hunde* cigars he liked to smoke.

Some curious recent research at the University of Chicago (McClintock and Pinto) has shown an interesting correlation between anosmia (loss of smell) and mortality. It would seem that not being able to smell is 'the canary in the coal mine of human health': it is not that loss of smell leads to death, it may be that loss of turnover of olfactory cells indicates a loss of regenerative potential elsewhere in the body.

The Importance of Being an Agoraphobe
[*Times Literary Supplement*, 2001]
It is perhaps slightly impertinent to end this 'obit' of a distinguished medical scientist on a note from Francis Bacon, who seems to have been utilitarian *avant la lettre* and might have disapproved of the virtuoso curiosity displayed by Petr Skrabanek, but modern society seems to be caught in the jaws of an only seemingly paradoxical question: how reasonable is it to be rational? In other words, where do human curiosity and ingenuity tip over into science as mere mechanism and technique? 'Natural science gives us an answer to the question of what we must do if we wish to master life technically', wrote Max Weber, the great German sociologist. 'It leaves quite aside, or assumes for its purposes, whether we should and do wish to master life technically and whether it ultimately makes sense to do so.'

The Human Position

[*PN Review*, 1997, as 'The Human Position: An Essay on Technology and Suffering']

More recently I read Pascal Quignard's *Les desarçonnés*, the seventh volume of his *Last Kingdom* series, and yet another book in which he combines aphorism, philosophical excursus, observation and novelistic fragment. His book is a meditation on what it means to fall, specifically out of the saddle. For that is the meaning of the verb *desarçonner*: to be unseated from the *arçon*, an old French word for the saddle tree. Trees and forests have supplied humans with primordial metaphors for notions of continuity and structure: there is the Tree of Life, and also the family tree; and there is the saddle tree, which at one point in human history offered a man a seat as high as he could get in the world. Now, in an age when everyone is a pedestrian (or cocooned in his car), the posture of a man on his high horse seems slightly ridiculous.

Nevertheless, Montaigne wrote that if he were allowed to choose, he would 'prefer to die in the saddle rather than in [his] bed, away from home and far from his folk'. ('On vanity'.) He had several experiences during his life of falling from his horse, one of them almost fatal. Quignard—no doubt thinking of Saul on the road to Damascus and his redressment after his episode of postural hypotension as Paul—is fascinated by the central role played by this experience of falling from a horse: he offers the expression *être desarçonné* as a humbler synonym for the experience of depression.

The philosopher Friedrich Nietzsche, who rode horses in his writings and imagined he was a centaur, saw a painting of a horse by Van Dyck that made him happy, but lost his mind when he saw the actual misery of a maltreated drayhorse in a Turin street.

Emergent Properties

[*Quadrant*, essay-review of Simon Winchester's biography *Joseph Needham and the writing of Science and Civilisation in China*, 2009]

Many of the 'characters' who emerged in British intellectual life around the Second World War—Ludwig Wittgenstein and Isaiah Berlin to name another two—wouldn't get anywhere near a professorship today; and I suspect Needham, with his dramatic switch from embryology to sinology would be treated with disdain too. As the Master said: 'A man who can study for three years without giving a thought to his career is hard to find.' (Confucius, Analect 8.12.) Much of this has to do with the 'professionalisation' of the academy, in which modes of thought have been condensed into a technique (or, worse, a mode of rhetoric), and little credence is given to originality or what used to be called 'amateurism'. Needham, for all his brilliance (and he is one of the few western scholars honoured by the Chinese), had something of the perpetual adolescent about him. Yet it may well be that the openness of adolescence is as close a quality as we have in our society to universality.

A Mining Town in Australia
[*PN Review*, 1998 as 'A Letter from Australia']
The all-enveloping boredom of outback Australia—where the immensity is so enormous and the horizon the same in every direction (a kind of abyss laid out flat)—is such as to take on a metaphysical dimension. The traveller might think to find there the ennui that Blaise Pascal thought was the condition proper to staying in one's room.

In fact, outback Australia is full of enterprising characters and a grittiness of truly surrealistic appeal, quite aside from the animal life. For fully five years after returning to Europe from Broken Hill, I had regular dreams of living in the town again; my wife and I are still in touch with friends we made during our year there. That said, Broken Hill was the quintessential Australian 'company town', with a single large employer able to hire and fire at will and despoil large tracts of the town, especially in the lee of the lead tailings.

I ought to add that had I had sufficient resilience to battle it out more directly with the forces changing the profession I wouldn't have written this book.

Lamplighters and Lucefactors
[*PN Review*, 1996, as a review of John Carey's anthology *The Faber Book of Science*]
The genial Paul Dirac (1902–1984), one of the key theorists of quantum mechanics and creator of an entirely new physical field theory which predicted the existence, in 1931, of antimatter, criticised Robert Oppenheimer for his interest in poetry. 'The aim

of science is to make difficult things understandable in a simpler way; the aim of poetry is to state simple things in an incomprehensible way. The two are incompatible.' (Kragh, *Dirac: A Scientific Biography*, 1990). Dirac's quip aside, we seem to have a powerful need to describe and interpret human functions in the terms of our inventions which take their place, and those tools in terms of the human functions that they replace. This used to be solely the domain of imaginative writers, but now scientists commonly indulge in acts of metaphoric transference, suggesting that not just body parts have machine-like qualities but the mind itself. This is not an innocent procedure, but one laden with consequences, as Raymond Tallis, for one, has shown in his many books.

Machine Made of Words
[*British Medical Journal*, 1998, as 'Biomedical Translation; and *The Linguist*, 1998, as 'Transcoding Technical 'Babble'']
Michel Serres in *Eclaircissements*, his interview book with Bruno Latour, adds: 'May I point out that each of my books describes a relationship, often expressed by a sole preposition? *Inter-ference*, for the spaces and times that are *between*; *communication* or *contract* for the relation expressed by the preposition *with*; *translation* for *across*; the *para-site* for *beside*... and so on. *Statues* is my counterbook and asks the question: What happens in the absence of relations?' Serres sees it as his lifework to devise the 'maritime map' of these 'spaces and times that precede any thesis (meaning position)'.

In her book *English: Meaning and Culture* (2006) Anna Wierzbicka provides a fascinating account of how specifically English-bound 'fairness' is: far from being a universal it is a unique creation of the culture that also associates coolheadedness with reasonableness, both of them questionable assumptions for many other cultures and languages.

And the famously gloomy French essayist and chronicler E. M. Cioran put in a good word for translators in *Aveux*: 'I have known obtuse writers, even stupid ones. One the other hand, the translators I have managed to approach were more intelligent, and more interesting that the authors they translated. After all, it takes more reflection to translate than "to create".'

The Poison Tree
[*Quadrant*, 2014, as 'The Upas Tree']
This essay, which ventures from Glasgow to Norilsk via Ambon, offers a glimpse of my more recent activity as a primary health care consultant in south-east Asia. There is almost no trace of Rumphius on Ambon, which I visited in 2014, other than his tomb and the forbidding hulks of some of the Dutch forts that provided protection for the assets of his employer, the Dutch East India Company (VOC). Somehow, in spite of its lengthy gothic shadow, the upas tree, which gave me my title, has vanished from the romantic herbarium. Three centuries after his death, most of Rumphius' work has finally appeared in English thanks to the heroic endeavours of the late Professor Beekman following his retirement from the University of Massachusetts, and the sponsorship of Yale University Press. There are some attentive references to Rumphius' presence on Ambon in the distinguished Dutch novel by Maria Dermoût, published in English as *The Ten Thousand Things* (*De Tienduizend Dingen*, 1958).

Stendhal's Syndrome
[*British Journal of General Practice*, 2010]
According to one medical journal which took Stendhal's syndrome more at face value than I do here, travelling is a 'concentrate of stressors': psychotic disorders are apparently at cause in ten to twenty percent of tourists requiring medical evacuation. For those who prefer their voyaging in the armchair Stendhal is a boon travelling companion, not least the account of the trip he made around the Midi in 1837–38 and published as *Mémoires d'un Touriste*: he claimed it was a book for the provincial 'who still does not know that everything is life is a comedy'. The anecdote in 'A Taste of Bitter Almonds' came from its pages.

Aqueous ammonium carbonate—*sal volatile*, or smelling salts—was widely used in Victorian times, and is still used in some sports, to arouse consciousness. I remember a rather stiff teacher at my primary school who surreptitiously took out her little bottle from a breast-pocket and sniffed on it whenever her class of beastly eight-year-olds had become too much for her.

The War of Eye and Ear

[*The Lancet*, 2002, as a filler; and *PN Review* 2008, as an expanded essay, 'On the Senses as Perceptual Systems']

It should be said that Aristotle, in contrast to Plato, doubted that our eyes emitted anything at all, surmising that they passively receive the radiation of visible objects: this is the intromission theory of vision. It took Emmanuel Kant to revive extramission, but in the form of projected mental images of the empirical world.

It was only when I finished this article that I realised I had written a variant on the classic Athens versus Jerusalem essay on the origins of European civilisation. In the story of the burning bush, Moses shields his eyes so as not to catch sight of God's face: in refusing sight, he begins to hear the voice. And this notion of figural emptiness as a recipient for divine instruction never leaves Western civilisation: Hegel's philosophy is essentially an instruction for us to become, ontologically, enemies or at least aliens to ourselves.

The obsession with sight and sightedness is by no means limited to the sciences. The avant-garde artist and Bauhaus theorist László Moholy-Nagy talked about 'the hygiene of the optical', and suggested that creative use of the camera would, by cleansing vision and educating the subconscious, make amends for the depredations of capitalism. By contrast, Emmanuel Levinas' phenomenology gave primacy to the ear over the eye; he also attributed expressivity to the face, which could 'speak' before the mouth opened. In a late poem, Paul Celan expresses most concisely the attention to the other person that I was trying to advocate. '…hör dich ein / mit dem Mund.' (Listen in / with your mouth.)

If anything, these days, it's not just that doctors don't have the time to listen properly to their patients; they don't touch them much either. Machines do the diagnostic work so much more expeditiously.

Under the Magic Mountain

[*Lapham's Quarterly*, 2009, as 'Course of Illness: A Reappraisal of Thomas Mann's *The Magic Mountain*']

In her book of recollections *Meine ungeschriebenen Memoiren* (1974) Thomas Mann's wife Katia raised the possibility that the ill-defined health problem that had afflicted her after the birth of her fourth child (she had six children altogether) and led her Munich doctors to send her for months at a time to various fashionable retreats in the Swiss valleys—which included Dr Friedrich Jessen's Waldsanatorium in Davos—might 'have cleared up of itself'.

Or perhaps she had never had 'incipient' TB in the first place? Four years before she published her memoir, a lung specialist, Professor Christian Virchow, had looked at the well-preserved X-ray films from 1912 and told her that for all his 'intensive study there was no finding to suggest incipient tuberculosis'. In their biography *Frau Thomas Mann* (2003) Inge and Walter Jens reveal that Katia Mann wouldn't countenance any talk of a diagnostic error—'implying of course that The Magic Mountain novel would in significant parts have been based on a medical mistake'.

Whether a mistake or not, it doesn't in the least detract from the novel, which at one level explores all the possibilities of human wilfulness and perversity, and not always those generated by 'illnesses'. German doctors don't contradict their rich patients who have private insurance today, quite the reverse; and there is no reason to imagine they did in the 1910s either. A sarcastic letter-writer once termed this 'opulence-based' medicine.

Katia Mann died in 1980, aged ninety-seven.

The Life and Times of Ernst Weiss
[*Times Literary Supplement*, 2010, essay-review of Ernst Weiss' novel *Georg Letham:Arzt und Mörder*, translated by Joel Rotenberg]
I have written about Ernst Weiss elsewhere, and the rather sensationalist account of Hitler's 'conversion experience' under hypnosis in 1918 as described in his novel *The Eyewitness* (1963). It has to be said that for want of reliable documentary testimony this episode receives only glancing mention in the major biographies, although Hitler seems to refer to it himself in *Mein Kampf*. Whatever happened in Dr Forster's Brandenburg clinic, the Führer's behaviour was more obviously influenced by another physician entirely: his 'Leibarzt' or personal physician, the shadowy Theodor Gilbert Morell, whom most of the Nazi leadership dismissed (with good reason) as a quack. In addition to cocaine eyedrops, the 'tonic' injections of the 'Reichsspritzenminister' are known to have included methamphetamine, strychnine and other dubious substances.

The classic text on the dilemmas presented by yellow fever in the colonial development of central America can be found in François Delaporte's *The history of yellow fever: an essay on the birth of tropical medicine*, in its able translation by Arthur Goldhammer (1991).

Parasites
[*Northern Review*, 1996]
Years later after writing this essay, which reflects on my experience of studying parasitology at the London School of Hygiene and Tropical Medicine, I discovered amongst the brilliant aphorisms and observations of the Viennese physician and writer Arthur Schnitzler (volume 5 of his *Collected Works*) the following entry: 'Notions such as "parasitizing", "corrupting", "extorting" are generally understood solely in a material sense. But aren't there parasites attached to our being, ones much worse than those which help themselves to earthly goods? Aren't there forms of corruption more subtle and even more underhand than those which exploit money and values? And aren't the worst forms of blackmail those which attack our feelings or attempt to?' It might even be thought, following on from Schnitzler, who was writing well before the Second World War, that our culture has become parasitic, feeding on its own past, and not always in an edifying way.

As for the hybrid nature of human beings, it would seem that at least part of our DNA has been picked up from seemingly utterly alien species: a study in *Genome Biology* suggests that the ABO antigen system which codes for the basic blood groups is bacterial in origin, the gene associated with fat mass derives from marine algae and that the group of genes which synthesize hyaluronic acid, an intracellular binding substance, was captured from fungi.

Twenty years ago, only a few specialists were interested in the gut: now the microbiome, the ecology of symbiotic microorganisms that inhabits our inner body space, is one of the trendiest topics around, and not just because antibiotic resistance has become medicine's 'global warming' equivalent. The unsung symbionts of our gut provide us with a not insignificant part of our calorific intake, manufacture vitamins and co-factors and protect us against pathogens.

Index of Names

d'Agoty, Jacques Gautier, 12
Alberti, Leon Battista, 227
Amis, Martin, 191
Anaxagoras, 226
Aristotle, 196, 204, 226
Ashbery, John, 206
Auden, Wystan Hugh, 43, 62, 65,
150, 152–58, 161–3, 178, 189,
191, 197, 232, 254
Auerbach, Erich, 230
Austen, Jane, 68

Babel, Isaac Emmanuilovich, 102,
139
Bacon, Francis, 16, 150, 183, 192,
193, 228, 258
Bacon, Reginald Hugh Spencer,
138–39
Baker, Nicholson, 102, 139
Bakhtin, Mikhail Mikhailovich, 229
de Balzac, Honoré, 19, 121, 214
Barnes, Julian, 224
Barthes, Roland, 127, 220
Baudelaire, Charles, 9
Baudrillard, Jean, 60, 132, 273
Bauer, Grete, 107
Bayley, John, 215
Bean, Charles Edwin Woodrow,
179
Beebe, William, 190
Beekman, Eric Montague, 211–13,
281
Benjamin, Walter, 45, 102, 110, 157,
162, 187, 205–6, 226
von Benkendorff, Alexander, 215
Bentham, Jeremy, 62, 67, 209, 232
Bernard, Claude, 19, 121
Beuys, Joseph, 12–15
Bevan, Aneurin, 149
Beyle, Marie-Henri (see Stendhal)
Blake, William, 214, 216, 234
Boccioni, Umberto, 12
Boehme, Jakob, 133
Bonaparte, Napoleon, 142, 218–19
Booth, Charles, 81
Borges, Jorge Luis, 7
Born, Max, 189
Boswell, James, 136–37, 223

Brecht, Bertolt, 102, 113, 134, 142,
240, 268, 277
Brod, Max, 98, 101, 102, 109, 110,
115, 116
Brooks, Mel, 254
Browne, Thomas, 7, 16, 121
Buber, Martin, 103
Buffon, Georges-Louis-Marie
Leclerc, 121
Bulgakov, Mikhail Afanassievitch, 96
Burke, Edmund, 96
Burns, Robert, 63
Burton, Robert, 39
Butler, Hubert, 96

Callimachus of Cyrene, 221
Calvino, Italo, 189
Camporesi, Piero, 141
Canetti, Elias, 42, 44, 110, 131–32,
135
Carey, John, 187–88, 189, 191–93,
195, 197–99
Carrère, Emmanuel, 71–72, 73,
75–78, 274
Cavell, Stanley, 233
Céline, Louis-Ferdinand, x, 24, 198,
271
Ceronetti, Guido, 30, 143
Chamberlain, Joseph, 263
Charcot, Jean-Martin, 23
de Chardin, Teilhard, 229
Checkland, Sydney, 208–9
Chekhov, Anton Pavlovich, 79–96,
180
Chekhov, Nikolai Pavlovich, 81
Chesterton, Gilbert Keith, 38
Chomsky, Avram Noah, 119
Cobb, Richard, 18
Cockeram, Henry, 121
Coleridge, Samuel Taylor, 196–97,
209, 210, 214
Conrad, Joseph, 84, 93, 138
Constant, Benjamin, 150
Corbin, Alain, 141
Coué, Émile, 28, 271
Curie, Marie, 188
Curie, Pierre, 188

Dalgarno, George, 187
Dali, Salvador, 11
Dampier, William, 176
Danby, Francis, 214
Dante Alighieri, 88, 92, 124, 145, 184, 229
Darwin, Charles, 21, 122, 135
Darwin, Erasmus, 188, 214
Davies, Norman, 230
Davy, Humphry, 210
Dawkins, Richard, 125, 189, 191
Defoe, Daniel, 210
Descartes, René, 231, 273
Dick, Philip Kindred, 71
Dickens, Charles, 154, 210, 214
Disney, Walt, 195
Dostoevsky, Fyodor Mikhailovich, 65, 76, 184, 185, 220
Douglas, Mary, 16
Duchenne de Boulogne, Guillaume-Benjamin, 135
Dürer, Albrecht, 12, 227
Durkheim, Émile, 8
Dymant, Dora, 101

Eddington, Arthur Stanley, 187, 199
Eisenstein, Sergei Mikhailovich, 102
Elias, Norbert, 226
ben Eli'ezer, Israel, 103
Elliott, Carl, 33, 65–67, 271, 273
Engels, Friedrich, 261

Fabre, Jean-Henri, 188
Fenton, James, 121–22, 196
Ferreri, Marco, 60
Fischart, Johann, 138
Flaubert, Gustave, 4, 121, 140, 273
Fletcher, Horace, 100
Fontana, Felice, 8
Fontane, Theodor, 66
Forster, Edmund, 254, 283
Foucault, Michel, 107, 246
Fragonard, Jean-Honoré, 12
Freud, Sigmund, 23, 27, 43, 50, 58, 61, 66, 112, 142, 147, 189, 222, 253
Fuller, Richard Buckminster, 122

Gadda, Carlo Emilio, 192, 206
Galen of Pergamon, 57, 270
Galilei, Galileo, 149, 188

Galkin-Vraskoy, Mikhail Nikolayevich, 85, 89
Garin-Mikhailovsky, Nikolai Georgievich, 85
Gerhardi, William, 95
Gibson, William, 126
Gide, André, 18
Girard, René, 76
Gish, Lillian, 176
Gladstone, William, 52
von Goethe, Johann Wolfgang, 9, 103, 121, 157, 159, 192, 218, 221, 240–41, 250
Goffman, Erving, 67
Gogol, Nikolai Vasilievich, 84, 92, 137–38, 144, 145
Gombrowicz, Witold, 76
Goncharov, Ivan Alexandrovich, 179
Gonzalez-Crussi, Frank, 7, 9
Gould, Stephen Jay, 188
Goupillières, Roger, 18
Graham, William Sydney, 232
Green, Henry, 53
Greene, Graham, 18

Hagens, Günther, 10–16, 270
Hauptmann, Gerhart, 247
Hauser, Kaspar, 73
Healy, David, 35–36, 271
Heller, Erich, 102, 106
Helman, Cecil, 55
Hemingway, Ernest, 50
Heraclitus, 143, 226
Herodotus, 221
Herz, Rachel, 140
Hesiod, 59
Hill, Austin Bradford, 149
Hippocrates of Kos, 26, 29, 226
Hirst, Damien, 50, 270
Hitler, Adolf, 29, 31, 111, 115, 256, 258, 261, 283
Hobbes, Thomas, 90
von Hofmannsthal, Hugo, 192
Hogarth, William, 7, 110
Hoggart, Richard, 139–40
d'Holbach, Paul-Henri Thiry, 63
Holbein, Hans, 220
Holtzmann, Bettyann, 244
Holub, Miroslav, 50, 150, 159, 191, 196, 198, 267
Hopkins, Claude C., 132

Horton, Richard, 36
Hughes, Robert, 91
Hughes, Ted, 196
Hugo, Victor, 183, 229
von Humboldt, Alexander, 110
Hume, David, 94, 147, 148, 233
Hunter, William, 8
Huxley, Thomas Henry, 188

Ibsen, Henrik Johan, 105
Inturissi, Louis, 223

Jack, Ian, 133–4
Jesenská, Milena, 106, 275
Johnson, Mark, 205
Johnson, Samuel, 63, 121, 136–37, 214, 223
Jones, Chuck, 129
Joseph II of Austria, 8
Josipovici, Gabriel, 111–12
Jouvet, Louis, 18, 22, 30, 271
Joyce, James, 43, 47, 121, 233, 274
Jung, Carl Gustav, 222, 251

Kafka, Franz, 42, 56, 59, 97–117 *passim*, 133, 155, 156, 179–80, 187, 189, 191, 195, 196, 199, 223, 252, 257
Kafka, Hermann, 98, 101
Kafka, Ottla, 97, 100, 101, 117
Kant, Immanuel, 148, 220, 240, 282
Karloff, Boris, 11
Kekulé, Friedrich August, 189
Kemble, Francis Anne, 174
Kennan, George, 95
Kepler, Johann, 169, 195
Kevorkian, Jack, 50
Kierkegaard, Søren, 115, 272
Kirmayer, Laurence, 35
von Kleist, Heinrich, 103, 174, 248
Klopstock, Robert, 112, 113, 275
Koch, Robert, 99
Kocher, Emil Theodor, 253
de Kooning, Willem, 133
Kouchner, Bernard, 70
Kramer, Peter, 35
Kraus, Karl, 38, 118–19, 129

Ladmiral, Luc, 69, 73
Laing, Ronald David, 78
Lakoff, George, 205

Lawrence, David Herbert, 247
Le Corbusier (Jeanneret-Gris, Charles-Édouard), 183
Lec, Stanisław Jerzy, 118
Leenhardt, Maurice, 8
Lefranc, Guy, 18
Lehmann, Heinz, 34
Leibniz, Gottfried Wilhelm, 38, 187
Leiris, Michel, 15
de Lempicka, Tamara, 255
Lenin (Ulianov, Vladimir Ilyich), 84
Leopardi, Giacomo, 145
Leopold II of Belgium, 84
Levi, Primo, 123, 188
Lévi-Strauss, Claude, 199
Levinas, Emmanuel, 41, 48
Levitan, Isaak Ilyich, 86
Li Bing, 166
Lichtenberg, Georg Christoph, 32, 67, 120
Linnaeus (von Linné), Carl, 121, 212
Löwy, Siegfried, 98–101
Lu Gwei-djen, 165, 169, 170
Luther, Martin, 13, 138
Lynch, Thomas, 49–53, 272–73

MacDiarmid, Hugh (Grieve, Christopher Murray), 197, 266
McLuhan, Herbert Marshall, 230, 234
Magherini, Graziella, 221
Malaparte, Curzio (Suckert, Kurt Erich), 132, 270
Malcolm, Janet, 95, 275
Malthus, Robert, 188
Mandelstam, Osip Emilyevich, 122, 132, 138–39, 189, 121, 167
Mann, Heinrich, 240
Mann, Thomas, 27, 84, 236–51 *passim*, 253, 256, 257, 282–83
Mao Zedong, 167, 169
Marar, Ziyad, 62–64, 67, 273
Marcus, Ben, 126
Marcuse, Herbert, 250
Margulis, Lynn, 122
Márquez, Gabriel García, 178
Mars-Jones, Adam, 140
Marx, Karl, x, 31, 11, 273
Massie, Allan, 210
Maxwell, James Clerk, 188
Mechin, Colette, 56, 273

Medawar, Peter Brian, 193
Mérimée, Prosper, 3
Mesmer, Franz Anton, 27
de la Mettrie, Julien Offray, 62–64
Miller, William Ian, 141
Mitford, Jessica, 52
Molière (Poquelin, Jean-Baptiste), 20, 22, 32, 127
Monro, Alexander, 10
de Montaigne, Michel, 67, 141, 163, 278
Morgan, Edwin, 196
Müller, Johannes, 100
Munthe, Axel, 22–23
Musil, Robert, ix, 192–93, 197–99
Mussolini, Benito, 27

Nabokov, Vladimir Vladimirovich, 40, 89, 93, 137, 144, 190
Naipaul, Vidiadhar Surajprasad, 191
Needham, Dorothy Moyle, 165
Needham, Joseph, 164–71, 213, 278
Newmark, Peter, 201
Newton, Isaac, 189, 192, 196, 197
Nicholson, Jack, 18
Nietzsche, Friedrich, 15, 28, 43, 59, 62, 67–68, 77, 104, 110, 111, 139, 143–44, 156, 158, 215, 230, 247, 260, 267, 268, 278
Nobel, Alfred, 124
Novalis (von Hardenberg, Georg Philipp Friedrich), 237

Orwell, George (Blair, Eric), 38, 119, 140, 174, 189, 201, 204
Osler, William, 56

Paré, Ambroise, 8
Parens, Erik, 34
Pasteur, Louis, 23, 82, 198, 261
Pavlov, Ivan Petrovich, 82
Peacock, Thomas Love, 196
Perec, Georges, 77, 126, 193
Peter the Great, 12
Picken, Laurence, 168
Pirandello, Luigi, 17
Plato, 26, 37, 57, 185, 209, 225, 226, 229, 282
Poe, Edgar Allan, 133
Poincaré, Henri, 93
Ponge, Francis, 196

Pope, Alexander, 68
Popper, Karl, 147
Pressburger, Giorgio, 134, 135
Priestley, John Boynton, 188
Pritchett, Victor Sawdon, 56, 142
Proctor, Robert, 29
Proust, Marcel, 4, 24, 44–45, 47, 140, 169, 188, 189, 213, 220
Pushkin, Alexander Sergeyevich, 215
Pythagoras of Samos, 231

de Quincey, Thomas, 86, 188

Rabelais, François, 57, 127, 227–34 passim
Raffles, Stamford, 214
Rasp, Charles, 175
Ravachol (Kœnigstein, François Claudius), 21
Reed, William, 256
Reich, Robert, 67
Rilke, Rainer Maria, 44, 138, 220, 232
Robertson, James, 210
Robertson, Robin, 51
de la Rochefoucauld, François, 62
Roentgen, Wilhelm Conrad, 189
Roget, Peter Marc, ix, 128
Romains, Jules, 17–32 passim, 271
Romand, Jean-Claude, 69–78 passim, 274
Rorie, David, 108
Rose, Nikolas, 237
Ross, Ronald, 188, 261
Roth, Joseph, 144, 253
Roth, Philip, 134
Rousseau, Jean-Jacques, 63, 67, 77, 114, 142, 218
Rowlandson, Thomas, 56, 110
Rumphius, George Eberhard, 211–14, 281
Ruskin, John, 214, 224
Ruysch, Frederik, 12

Sacks, Oliver, 189
de Sade, Donatien Alphonse François, 66, 114
Schemm, Hans, 29
Schnitzler, Julius, 253, 284
Scholem, Gershom, 110, 187, 226, 233

Schopenhauer, Arthur, 59
Schwartz, Karlene V., 122
Schweitzer, Albert, 78
Sebald, Winfried Georg, 220
Sewel, William, 212
Shakespeare, William, 88, 104, 121,
   196, 214, 228, 229, 231, 234–35,
   258
Shaw, George Bernard, 17, 22, 189
Simmel, Georg, 231
Skrabanek, Petr, 146–50, 277
Sloterdijk, Peter, 250
Smellie, William, 8
Smith, Zadie, 134
Snow, John, 29
Sontag, Susan, 239
Stalin, Joseph, 132, 139, 215
Stanley, Henry Morton, 84
Starobinski, Jean, 227
Steevens, George, 214
Stein, Marc Aurel, 166
Steiner, George, 169, 213, 230
Stendhal (Beyle, Marie-Henri), 3–5,
   63, 66, 144, 145, 218–25
Stern, Joseph Peter, 115
Sterne, Laurence, ix, x, 136, 199, 218
Stevenson, Robert Louis, 77
Straße, Hans, 100
Strauss, Emmanuel, 108
Süskind, Patrick, 141
Suvorin, Aleksey Sergeyevich, 79, 81,
   82, 85, 86, 89, 93–95
Sweeney, Matthew, 51
Swift, Jonathan, 38, 87, 88, 188, 204
Sydenham, Thomas, 119
Szasz, Thomas, 36

Tenner, Edward, 127
Theresa of Avila, 143
de Tocqueville, Alexis-Charles-Henri
   Clérel, 150

Tolstoy, Leo Nikolayevich, 21,
   81–84, 94, 138
Turgenev, Ivan Sergeyevich, 93
Twain, Mark, 28, 202, 223–24

Valverde, Juan, 11
Veblen, Thorstein, 65
Verne, Jules, 60, 184
Vesalius, Andreas, 9
da Vinci, Leonardo, 12, 155, 187,
   195, 224, 227
Voltaire (Arouet, François-Marie),
   229, 237

von Wackenfels, Wackher, 169
Wagenbach, Klaus, 97, 117
Wang Ling, 167
Waugh, Evelyn, 52
Weigand, Hermann, 236
Weil, Simone, 25, 28
Weinberger, Eliot, 131
Weiss, Ernst, 252–59
Wells, Herbert George, 183
Wilkins, John, 121
William of Ockham, 8
Williams, William Carlos, 190–91
Winchester, Simon, 166, 170, 278
Wittgenstein, Ludwig, 65, 82, 102,
   106, 139, 154, 186–87, 188, 192,
   231, 278
Wolfe, Tom, 64
Wolff, Kurt, 98
Wright, Jabez

Yeats, William Butler, 146, 197

Zamenhof, Ludwik Lejzer, 203
Zhou Enlai, 167
Zola, Émile, 24, 83, 86, 121, 189
Zummo, Gaetano, 8
Zweig, Stefan, 17, 30, 253